LAKE BLUFF PUBLIC LIBRARY

3 0401 0019 2412 9

S0-BFC-804

JUN – – 2014

Praise for Carolina Fröhlich

'Without you, we would not have got through this. He is now able to read against all the odds and he has regained his self-esteem; he is a much happier boy. Thank you.' *Lisa and David, Sussex*

'I want to congratulate you on your book. It's brilliant. I have just finished reading it. Most of your book is wisdom for any parent, not only for those with children who have dyslexia. Your book is already making a difference!' *Ophelia, Germany*

'Carolina's knowledge and empathy is evident from all angles. She is a role model for parents who want to preserve confidence and self-esteem in their children.' *Martin, London*

'This book is a comprehensive guide to recognising and understanding dyslexia and to supporting your children right through the educational system. I wish your book had been available when our now 14-year-old was going through hell. If I had had access to this several years ago, the earlier years stuff would have had more impact than anything I found at the time.' *Pam, London*

'Carolina has been very supportive throughout our journey of identifying our son's learning issues. This includes underachieving and executive functioning issues. We have been hard pushed to understand how this should be managed. Carolina has suggested strategies for home, and has helped us to understand how we can work with the school and teachers that are involved in our son's daily & school environment. Carolina is thorough, professional and can communicate in ways that parents can understand. She is able to pull from a wealth of resources and information. We really appreciate all the support she has offered to us and we are now seeing positive results at home and school. We are more confident in being able to manage our little boy appropriately and with less stress.' *Al, Netherlands*

LAKE BLUFF PUBLIC LIBRARY
123 Scranton Avenue
Lake Bluff, IL 60044

Dyslexia:

TIME FOR TALENT

– Early Years to University –

Dyslexia:

TIME FOR TALENT

The Ultimate Guide for Parents and Children

CAROLINA FRÖHLICH

Fröhlich Publishing Ltd
Arden, Peaslake Lane
Guildford, Surrey
GU5 9RL
United Kingdom

First published in 2014

Copyright © 2014 Carolina Fröhlich

ISBN 978-0-9566435-2-0

First Edition

All rights reserved. No part of this publication, including text and drawings, may be reproduced, stored in a retrieval system or transmitted, in any form or by any means, electronic, mechanical, photocopying, recording or otherwise, without the prior permission of the copyright holder. The author claims moral right under the Copyright, Design and Patent Act 1988.

Although the author and publisher have made every effort to ensure that the information in this book was correct at press time, the author and publisher do not assume and hereby disclaim any liability to any party for any loss, damage, or disruption caused by errors or omissions, whether such errors or omissions result from negligence, accident, or any other cause. This book is not intended as a substitute for the medical advice of physicians/doctors/psychologists. The reader should regularly consult a physician/doctor/psychologist in matters relating to his/her health, well-being and that of a child, particularly with respect to any symptoms that may require diagnosis or medical attention.

Contact the author: **www.carolinafrohlich.co.uk**

Illustrations by Dominique Sanson
Digital images by Carolina Fröhlich and Diana Bustamante

To my children,
Gemma and Alex

Contents

List of tables

Foreword

I am delighted to write the foreword to this timely and comprehensive book. Published to celebrate Dyslexia Awareness Week in the UK, there is also helpful advice and information at an *international* level for people in English-speaking schools across the world.

Carolina Fröhlich's views on dyslexia resonate perfectly with the training she received at the Helen Arkell Dyslexia Centre some years ago. The HADC motto is 'making the most of a difference' and this could well be the strap line for *Time for Talent*.

This comprehensive book celebrates the difference in style and learning that people with dyslexia bring to their worlds at home, school and in the workplace. Carolina speaks as a parent and as an educator as well as offering her own dyslexic perspective.

The book is accessible, informative and positive. It works right through the age range to adulthood and this journey of support is made credible by the many case studies showing dyslexia alongside co-existing difficulties. Refer to it as a complete book of recipes – some for now, some for later. Or, treat it like the road map that Carolina offers and get on with your journey wherever you are. The comprehensive nature of *Time for Talent* means that many holistic approaches are included for those who want to add these to their toolkit.

Parents of children with dyslexia will find *Time for Talent* invaluable; in fact I would suggest that there are excellent parenting strategies for parents of any children.

This is the ideal book for the multiple diversity of people who have dyslexia, and the multi-faceted people who care for them – something for everyone.

Bernadette McLean
Principal of the Helen Arkell Dyslexia Centre

Note from the author

Time for Talent encompasses a wealth of information about living with and triumphing over the day-to-day learning, social, behavioural and emotional challenges of dyslexia and other specific learning difficulties. When you have read it, I recommend keeping it handy as a reference guide when you are looking for answers to specific problems as and when they occur.

When I did my first round of editing in digital format, I found it very helpful to use text to speech software to listen to the book, and you can use the text-to-speech facility on eReaders as an alternative way to access the ebook version.

The paperback book is printed on cream-coloured paper to avoid the glare of reading black print on a white background. I have purposely left-justified the paragraphs to make keeping one's place easier. I have used Century Gothic, a sans-serif font (which has a rounded 'a' and does not have the 'ticks' and 'tails' at the end of strokes that makes reading easier for those who have dyslexia).

This book is intended for parents in all English-speaking countries, including expats and homeschooling parents. In the case of homeschooling parents, I have generically referred to 'school' and 'classroom', which of course would be replaced with 'learning at home'. For grammatical consistency, I have referred to your child as 'he'; but please note that dyslexia is not gender specific and affects both males and females alike.

As education systems vary from country to country, I mainly refer to the system in the UK, with some references to the USA, Canada and Australia. Many countries still do not recognise dyslexia sufficiently and therefore may not have dyslexia awareness or best practice systems in place. If this is the case in your country, please take heart from this book and know what is possible – perhaps you can campaign for action in your school or country so that children do not need to suffer.

CF

The Author

Born in London, Carolina is a successful published author, international speaker, teacher and consultant to struggling parents and schools. She coaches and mentors parents and children from all over the world. She lectures and gives seminars in the United Kingdom and in British and American International schools worldwide.

Carolina's objective is to give parents and teachers of children with dyslexia a fundamental and systemic understanding of the implications of having 'learning difficulties'. She provides practical strategies and tools that work at home and school, to ensure children and parents find the right path of lifelong positive learning, in spite of a perceived learning 'disability'.

Carolina has dyslexia. Along with her many years of teaching children, Carolina is the parent of two children with dyslexia and dyspraxia. She overcame her own dyslexia, using her difficulties to inspire children. Carolina truly understands the daily challenges that children and their families face with respect to education, achievement and self-esteem. Her passion is for maximising children's potential and empowering parents.

Her Time for Talent personalised mentoring system is the result of Carolina's 20-year study of dyslexia and other learning difficulties, and many years teaching children with learning challenges and empowering parents. Her holistic and unique mentoring approach empowers parents to support their child.

Carolina is a qualified specialist teacher, educational assessor, lecturer and speaker in dyslexia and specific learning difficulties for primary, secondary and further education. She has a Postgraduate Certificate of Education (PGCE), specific learning difficulties qualifications and educational assessor qualifications from the British Psychological Society and Psychological Testing Centre. Her first degree is in Business Studies.

Acknowledgements

As I begin to reflect on the magnitude of writing this book, I am reminded that this project is the inspiration of many. I am enormously grateful to Ann Davies and Lynne Skinner for their eternal support and enthusiasm; Kim Richardson for living through dyslexia with me and our children; Martin for giving me the confidence to write this book; Jennifer Simpson, Carolyn Wilson and Bernadette McLean for being amazing dyslexia ambassadors and making a difference in our lives. My wonderful parents, friends and work colleagues: Aggie, Claudia, Caroline, John, Jenny, Pam, Max, Ophelia, Carla, Dominique, Diana and Judy. A big thank you to Lesley for editing this book – what a task!

Thank you kindly to the following organisations and individuals for giving me permission to cite their works: British Dyslexia Association, Potential Plus UK, British Psychological Society (Scottish Division), Dyspraxia Foundation, Mensa, Dr Linda Silverman and Dr Anna Wilson.

- To all the researchers and theorists who have discovered so much and continue to find new ways to help people with dyslexia.
- To all the teachers and special needs teachers: without your dedication, our children would not become the people they have the potential to be.
- To all the wonderful children I have had the privilege to teach: you are an inspiration.
- To all the amazing parents who have sought my help: you made me realise that this book needed to be written in this style.

And most of all, thank you to my darling children, Gemma and Alex, for your love, inspiration, encouragement, wisdom and for being born exactly who you are. Thank you for giving me the passion to help others with dyslexia, and for your support throughout the preoccupations with the challenges of writing. This book is dedicated to you.

PART ONE
Our Children and Dyslexia

Chapter 1
Introduction

Understanding our children's frustrations and
giving them the tools to blossom will give
them the confidence to reach their true
potential. We can help our children channel
their interests and talents and ignite the
passion within.

Carolina Fröhlich

Hi, my name is Carolina, and I am the proud mother of a
great daughter and son. When I found out my daughter
and then my son had dyslexia, I had never heard of this
'condition' and didn't even know that I had dyslexia. There
were few books on the subject and it was not widely discussed
within schools or among friends. I felt alone, frightened and
very frustrated!

As I learned more about dyslexia and specific learning
difficulties (known as SpLD or LD) and what my children were
going through, I retrained as a specialist teacher, so that I
could learn more about how to help my children get through
their education and their lives with dyslexia.

My aim in writing this book is to share my knowledge, my
story, and stories from other parents and their children, to make
you aware of the latest research and resources available to
help your children who have dyslexia. I will share, from my
knowledge and experience as a parent, teacher and a
woman with dyslexia, the many ways you can help your
children at school.

I will offer you successful, practical strategies for getting
your children through their years of education, to enable you to

short-cut the journey that can take many parents much longer to make.

Why not love the ten years of schooling? Why wait until school is over to begin feeling good about life? The key is to change our mind-set and open our hearts to explore, develop and understand new methods of learning. If you have a child with dyslexia, your main concern is discovering what you and the school can do to help. You'll need patience, love, and understanding of what your child is going through to find the help you and your child need.

Patience, love, and understanding of what your child is going through

Whatever your own school experience was like, this book will help you understand how your child can be helped to get the most out of his school years. Your child may even learn to enjoy school! If you are homeschooling your child, you will find this book essential if you suspect a learning difficulty.

Originally trained as a business consultant, I had never worked with children. One evening after my daughter had been diagnosed with dyslexia, I was helping her with maths homework. Gemma was frustrated and angry with herself because she couldn't understand the homework. 'I don't know how to do this maths work', she screamed, 'I have never seen it before in my life! It's not fair that my teacher gives me something I've never learned before!' I put my arms around her and we talked things through. When she had calmed down, we began to attack the page of questions. I later found out that the topic had been covered in class the previous day. I also learned that forgetting things is a common characteristic of dyslexia.

Forgetting things is a common characteristic of dyslexia

By the time I retrained as a specialist teacher at the Helen Arkell Dyslexia Centre, I had spent years supporting my children with their homework and trying to raise their levels of self-confidence. It was a hard road. My son or daughter would wrestle with trying to read and retain large amounts of information. Remembering this spelling or interpreting that maths problem caused repeated upsets.

Having two children with dyslexia, I thought I knew a lot about dyslexia already. But, sometimes, I couldn't understand why they were finding reading so difficult or homework so tough. I felt I needed specialist knowledge. What I learned on the teaching course opened my eyes and changed my whole perception of our problem.

Today, there is a greater understanding of dyslexia and this unique style of learning. But how unique is it, if more than 10% of us have dyslexia? Dyslexia is not an illness but a different way of thinking and processing information. A person with dyslexia uses different parts of the brain when processing the written or spoken word compared to a non-dyslexic. I gained new knowledge on the course that made me even more sympathetic to my children's frustrations and gave me a new appreciation of their learning challenges in the classroom. Nowadays, I help parents and children learn in fun ways using multisensory, kinaesthetic (hands-on), memorable techniques specifically designed to appeal to the way that people with dyslexia learn. These new ways are very successful, and I am passing them on to you.

Among the many skills I acquired, I learned about phonics (a sounds-based approach to reading), phonemes (units of sound) and decoding skills (making sense of the written word by recognising individual units of sounds). These skills were very different from the ones I had been using! In nursery school and reception class, our children were learning Letterland. I knew all the letter names and sounds and felt I was doing a good job helping them read. I didn't know that sounding out difficult words letter by letter was not the right way to break them down. No one had taught us parents how to teach our children to read. No one had taught us that there are 44 phonic sounds in the English language, not 26! No one had taught us how to blend sounds!

Raising any child may be instinctive for some but we weren't taught how at school. When my children and I were going through their years of schooling, I sometimes did not feel like the perfect parent, although I tried hard to keep calm and remain positive. I did not push my kids so hard that it wiped them out, as they needed time to relax and be kids. I simply encouraged and supported them at all times, ensuring that they did not give up, and showed them the massive potential that lay within.

My understanding of how Gemma and Alex learn best, and getting them the help they needed, have made them fully understand their strengths and challenges as young adults. Both have developed a sense of determination and inner confidence because we drew on their strengths and developed their weaknesses. They have relayed to me their own feelings and experiences about how uncomfortable they felt at school and what did not work for them. Now my children support *me* with their wonderful ideas for games for the children I help.

My kids are proud that I am able to help other children with dyslexia. Both offered many suggestions when I was writing this book. Their biggest recommendations were to remind parents and teachers to make learning creative and *fun*; to find out what children are good at and love doing; for teachers not to criticise pupils' mistakes so much; to give much more praise for effort; and to try to understand what children are going through.

The parents and children I support today can access a wealth of knowledge and be brought up to speed much more quickly because of this approach. Parents frequently thank me for helping their children, but also for supporting them too. We parents really do need support.

Did you know that approximately 40% of all millionaires have dyslexia or have learning difficulties?[1] They didn't achieve success in spite of dyslexia – they were often successful *because* of it. Journalist Ben Dowell states: 'Psychologists who analysed the mental make-up of business winners found learning difficulties are one of the most important precursors of financial success.'[2]

However, in spite of our resourcefulness, originality and successes, many successful adults with dyslexia give negative accounts of their time at school. Nowadays, more knowledge and support is available and children should not tolerate being miserable, put down or unsuccessful at school. Your child's school years need not be a struggle.

Discovering that your child has dyslexia does not have to be doom and gloom. It can be a great relief finding out your child has dyslexia because your child and you will finally understand WHY he has had difficulties all along, and that it has NOTHING to do with being 'stupid' or 'lazy' or having a severe 'disorder'.

When my children and I were finding our way through the system and getting to grips with the support and information available, it often seemed like a never-ending battle. This book will arm you with the appropriate tools and knowledge for your child's whole education at home, school, college and university, so that you can support to the best of your ability. There are many ways you can help your child. You just need to know what they are!

Hello, dyslexia!

Chapter 2
Personal stories

Aged eight, I still couldn't read, in fact, I was dyslexic and short-sighted. Only after a couple of terms did anyone think to have my eyes tested. But even when I could see, the letters and numbers made no sense at all.

Richard Branson, entrepreneur[3]

My children

Gemma is a smart, thoughtful, enthusiastic and resourceful young woman with an incredible singing voice. As a toddler, she was happy and bouncy and met all the expected childhood milestones. She loved drawing, creating things, making up plays and listening to stories. She had a wild imagination, she sang like a bird, but... she did not want to read.

Both my children reached all the expected childhood milestones

When our children were pre-school age, we regularly took them to a farm where they could feed the animals and learn about their habitats, environment and offspring. Some of the parents were already unconsciously stretching their children through questioning techniques: 'Do you think all birds put their eggs into an incubator to hatch?' 'So, why do you think the owl sleeps during the day?' It was a glorious learning experience for all, without the formalities of pen and paper. Our children were learning through fun.

The first warning bell rang when most of the children in the group were showing signs of reading words like pig, cow and hen, but Gemma was not. She found it taxing and was upset at not being able to read them, but I was a long way from fully comprehending that she had dyslexia. Something was wrong but I couldn't pinpoint the exact cause. Perhaps she couldn't see or hear the word properly? Our family doctor arranged for a barrage of tests, which revealed no sight or hearing problem.

No sight or hearing problem

In Reception year,[4] Gemma continued to be creative and enjoyed organising her friends and suggesting innovative games. She was inspiring – a caring leader – a people person. She enjoyed drawing and singing the letters of the alphabet. She could associate them with their corresponding animal pictures and she knew all the letter tunes by heart. She adored school.

At home, Gemma's bedroom was adorned with Jolly Phonics posters, Letterland friezes and tons of children's books. She loved choosing a book, turning the pages, browsing through it and discussing and predicting the story. Bedtime stories were a must.

By the start of Year 1, it was apparent that Gemma was struggling to remember her letter sounds to decode (sound out) words. I couldn't understand why when she clearly knew the names and sounds of all 26 letters of the alphabet. She still loved school, but not reading.

By Year 2,[5] her contagious enthusiasm had begun to fade. Some days she did not want to go to school. There were tears and tantrums. Something was amiss. She finally confessed that she felt 'stupid'. As a parent, your heart sinks when you hear that word.

After much discussion with her teacher, we identified that Gemma was struggling with her reading and thus losing confidence in her ability to read aloud in class and do class work. Consequently, her self-esteem was suffering and school was no longer fun. So, when she was seven, I took her for a diagnostic educational assessment.

School was no longer fun

Although I was nervous, taking Gemma to be assessed was the best thing I could have done. Within hours, we began to understand her challenges and her many strengths. Her

9

assessment diagnosed her with dyslexia and speech and language difficulties and she was referred to a speech and language therapist (SALT).

Alex

Meanwhile, my son Alex, who had never enjoyed nursery school, was about to start Reception year at a different school.

Alex is a smart, caring and energetic young man with a big zest for life. He is an innovative leader whose thirst for and retention of factual information is amazing. As a toddler, he was very happy, loved drawing and singing. He also reached all the expected childhood milestones.

At school, Alex was good at sport, his schoolwork seemed well above average, he was artistic and his long-term memory was amazing. I thought his thirst for knowledge would motivate him to become a voracious reader - but he did not like reading.

One day, a teacher in the learning support department at Alex's school approached me out of the blue, knowing I had a daughter with dyslexia. She asked if she might use Alex as a case study in her doctorate research on specific learning difficulties. He was interesting to her because of the potential hereditary links in dyslexia. I agreed but said that there was no point, as my son had not been flagged up as having any difficulties in class and was not even having learning support.

Around the same time, Alex's class teacher mentioned in passing after watching a school play that his class work had deteriorated over the previous two terms. I was appalled that she had left it so long without calling us in for a meeting. Nevertheless, I was grateful that she had at least said something – even though it was very late and in an inappropriate way.

Well, you can imagine what came next... the tests revealed Alex probably did have dyslexia. So the learning support teacher recommended we have a formal educational assessment.

A different set of dyslexic characteristics emerged

His assessment diagnosed Alex with dyslexia and dyspraxia (fine motor control issues responsible for handwriting and a variety of other coordination skills). He, too, was referred to a speech and language therapist. He, also, had difficulty with reading, spelling and language. With hindsight, I had noticed some signs, but they were a different set of dyslexic characteristics from the ones with which I had become familiar.

So, we found ourselves going through the whole process of having learning support again. Alex was less willing than Gemma to accept that he had a learning challenge, as he had witnessed her outbursts of frustration on several occasions. As a consequence, he was quite reluctant to attend his before-school extra support lessons. But we were blessed with wonderful learning support teachers who made him feel special and clever and, with their love and guidance, we were eventually able to coax Alex into attending extra lessons.

Around this time, Gemma started middle school, complete with her educational psychologist's report detailing her learning profile, together with her areas of strength and challenge. The school had a small, dedicated learning support department and was able to offer some pupils one-to-one support. I felt that not only would Gemma receive the support she needed, but that I would get guidance too!

'Mummy, mummy, mummy, I got 29% in my English exam!'

At her new school, Gemma had a caring teacher who worked with her twice a week for the next four years. This teacher's dedication to all the children with learning 'opportunities' was tireless and inspiring.

One day, when Gemma was eight, she came flying into the pickup room with a huge smile, skipping for joy and shouting, 'Mummy, mummy, mummy, I got 29% in my English exam!'

We had an amazing afternoon celebrating her success. My daughter's self-esteem was high; she was flying, and so was I.

Although I later found out the median mark in the class was 65%, what might constitute a low grade to some parents was an enormous check mark in the success column for our family.

His teacher had taken the trouble to get to know his strengths

Alex also had a fantastic learning support teacher who had taken the trouble to get to know his strengths and had built upon his skills. He soon grew to like her very much and reluctantly accepted the benefit of having learning support. He did not enjoy being withdrawn from timetabled lessons but, fortunately for Alex, a few other boys in his class were also receiving individual support, which took the pressure off him, as he was no longer the only one requiring special treatment.

As we acclimatised to the challenges and learned to overcome them, there was always room for laughter. Now, looking back, we laugh at ourselves and feel relieved that it is turning out all right. However, even after diagnosis and assessment, even with support classes and loving, dedicated teachers, and even with unfailing commitment and patience on your part, I can't promise it will be all sunshine and roses. There are plenty of pitfalls but I will guide you through them.

Our story at school ended happily, in that both children have eventually done well, despite the hair pulling and floods of tears over the years. My daughter is a sales executive for a technology company in London and was shortlisted out of 7,000 applicants for just 24 positions, and my son has just achieved a 2:1 in his second year at university studying advertising.

A big challenge I found with my children's dyslexia was its impact on their self-confidence and, consequently, the detrimental effect on their self-esteem. I did not meet many people who openly discussed their child's dyslexia and sometimes this made us feel we were the only ones going through difficult times. I urge you to share your stories, your experiences and your knowledge, so that we can pull together, and so that future generations do not have to endure the long, and sometimes fraught, lonely journey of having dyslexia at school.

Share your stories, your experiences and your knowledge, so that we can pull together

True stories

There is great comfort in knowing and understanding what other people do in similar situations to those in which we find ourselves. From time immemorial, people have formed groups, tribes and societies to share their stories, triumphs, failures and successes and to learn from one another. Over time, reading and writing became skills that were desirable for ordinary people rather than the elite. Until it became possible to teach all children to read and write, a condition such as dyslexia would have been very difficult to detect. The term 'dyslexia' was first conceived in 1887 by Rudolf Berlin, a German ophthalmologist.

Until a generation or two ago, it was still very difficult to get dyslexia diagnosed, and much less accommodated, in the modern school system. However, great strides have been made in recent years and now many schools and universities have structured support systems in place to offer special help to dyslexic students.

The situation continues to improve as scientists and educational specialists make advances in understanding the physiological aspects of the inner working of the human brain, and we continue to improve our understanding of how humans learn and of the many different forms that intelligence can take.

So, it is getting better all the time but, until it's a perfect world, perhaps you can take comfort in hearing other people's stories. Names have been changed to preserve their anonymity.

Mike and Mary

Sally was seven years old when Mike and Mary noticed that she was having a lot of difficulty learning. At first, they thought she had a poor work ethic and wasn't interested in school. Later, they learned she had dyslexia.

Their initial reaction was of guilt and fear. Mike and Mary thought they must have been doing something to cause the dyslexia (dyslexia is a difference in the way the brain functions). Sally's school was supportive from the start and offered testing.

Once a diagnosis was made, it provided learning support, and Sally was taught excellent coping strategies. As a result, Sally's daily life has not been seriously impacted by her dyslexia.

Mike and Mary work at making sure that Sally has the tools and techniques to overcome her dyslexia. She particularly experiences short-term memory difficulties. They are confident that she has accepted her challenges and is using her techniques to work through them. The hardest part of finding out that she had dyslexia was trying to answer her question, 'Why?' At the time, they wished they had realised how common dyslexia is, as it would have made answering the question a little easier. No one else in Mike or Mary's family has dyslexia to their knowledge.

Mike and Mary have a strong belief in Sally. Their advice for other parents facing a similar situation is:

> 'Accept, support and fight for whatever help you can get and do not let anyone tell you that your child is not going to be successful.'

John

Jack was six when John realised that his son was not reading at the same level as other kids his age. He was also having a lot of trouble remembering things he had just been told. While Jack was still young, John assumed this was a natural immaturity all children go through, until he noticed that other kids were processing similar instructions from their parents without difficulty. When dyslexia was diagnosed, John had no idea how to begin dealing with it, or what obstacles lay ahead. John was worried about the long-term impacts that dyslexia would have on Jack's life.

Jack's school was supportive to a degree, and John says that he learned to work within 'their box'. Mostly, he learned to work with Jack so that Jack was not overwhelmed. John says he stopped to think carefully about every question he posed or task he asked Jack to do so as not to confuse him with complex lists or a complicated series of questions. When Jack was overwhelmed, he had a tendency to get upset, so John was careful to avoid putting Jack in situations that would provoke him.

It hurt to watch Jack struggle with remembering how to do his homework when he was tired after a long day of trying very hard at school. John was tired after work too. Finding the energy to deal with the demands of supporting and helping Jack was exhausting, yet John knew that, unless he came up with the inner strength to help out, Jack would suffer in the long term.

Thankfully, Jack's wonderful personality has been an asset in helping him cope with his dyslexia and the challenges it has brought. Jack is laid back and easy going and has a witty outlook on life that brings pleasure to those around him, especially his dad. John has never been officially diagnosed with dyslexia, but remembers having similar experiences to Jack's.

John's advice is that, even though each child is different:

> 'There is a lot to be learned by communicating with other parents of dyslexic children and sharing your experiences. You will get ideas and also give others ideas about things that are working for you.'

Sarah

Sarah's reaction on finding out that her son, Jay, has dyslexia, is one that probably sums up most parents' reactions:

> 'How do I deal with this?' 'Where do I start?'

Jay was only four years old when Sarah noticed that he was having difficulty learning. At primary school, his dyslexia was not picked up, and it was not until he was 11 that he was officially diagnosed.

Sarah worried about the long-term effects on Jay's self-confidence and on his overall prospects in life. He struggled endlessly with his homework and had trouble even getting started on it. Anything that required putting pen to paper was a major challenge for him.

However, his emotional intelligence was high and he always considers his actions carefully and the impact they will have on others. He has proved to have a resilient personality and great perseverance, which went in his favour on many occasions.

Along with his resilience, which Sarah sometimes thinks of as stubbornness, Jay has proven to be very hard working indeed since he started getting help at his new school. Now, he has stopped setting himself unattainable goals and has learned coping strategies to manage his dyslexia.

Sam and Julie

Julie and Sam discovered that Peter was having trouble in school when he was about eight years old. Peter had always been extremely bright, especially in maths. He was great at the computer and picked things up really fast. He also excelled in science. Julie mentioned that Peter has extremely sensitive hearing and can be 'easily annoyed by sounds that she cannot hear'. Julie and Sam thought his teacher that year was just not very good and attributed Peter's growing restlessness to the fact that he was not being stretched academically in school.

Before his diagnosis, he was unruly, always restless and prone to throwing tantrums. He was bored in class, and he exhibited bullying behaviour, which Julie thinks was a defence mechanism, as he also seemed to have an underlying fear even as he was bullying other kids. The family reached a turning point when the school informed Sam and Julie that Peter was being expelled for being 'restless, having a short concentration span and having constant squabbles with his classmates'. He was simply too disruptive to keep in school. The headmaster recommended sending Peter to a private specialist school. Peter's parents were left feeling completely abandoned by the school system and out on a limb.

No one in their family had ever been diagnosed with a learning disorder before. The expensive school that the headmaster recommended was for severe learning disorders (which had *nothing* to do with dyslexia!) Not knowing what else to do, they decided to enrol him in the school. As soon as he started there, they realised they had made a big mistake. Peter was still not doing well, and he got himself into even more trouble. Peter's parents responded by taking him out of that school and putting him back into a mainstream state school, but one that understood dyslexia.

After their ordeal, and with a strong belief in their own son, Sam and Julie decided to completely play down Peter's dyslexia and didn't want him to be treated differently in the classroom. He leaves the class periodically for literacy support lessons, but otherwise does everything the other children do and seems much happier now. His reading is improving and he is doing well at his cursive handwriting.

A supportive school can make a tremendous difference to your child's well-being and self-esteem

Julie and Sam learned that a supportive school can make a tremendous difference to a child's well-being and self-esteem. If your child is in a school that is not especially supportive of children with dyslexia, the road can be much, much harder. Their advice to parents is to ask the school about its special needs policy and what level of support it can offer to children with dyslexia. Then they recommend that parents get counselling on the subject. Julie had this to say about their counselling:

> 'Peter's father and I both went for a few months to get counselling in dyslexia; the advice we had was priceless!'

Sam and Julie's strategy for helping Peter was to offer praise for even the slightest improvement or achievement, whether it was an improvement in his everyday life at home or a step forward in something he was learning at school. Their strategies for helping him, together with the education they received themselves through counselling, have been so successful that they really don't notice his dyslexia very much anymore. Its impact on family life has been greatly lessened now that he has a supportive school environment as well as a nurturing home environment.

Julie says she feels extremely relieved now that Peter is getting incredible support for his dyslexia, and he is getting on much better now. Julie can't believe the amount of progress

Peter has made in a short time. She really admires Peter because he has had to cope with so much more than other kids and has gone through some very difficult situations at school, but is coming out successfully at the other end. Julie believes this experience has built Peter up to be strong.

Jo and Maria

Maria noticed that her daughter Laura, aged five, was having trouble remembering simple things and experiencing difficulty with hand-to-eye coordination, and brought it to the attention of Laura's teacher. Maria had two older children and so she thought she had a good frame of reference for knowing whether Laura was on track for her age. But Laura's teacher refused to acknowledge that there was a problem and told Maria that she should not measure Laura's progress against other children, even siblings. The teacher told Maria to stop being so pushy with Laura and allow her to develop in her own good time. Maria retreated, feeling duly reprimanded, but inside she still had a niggling feeling that all was not quite right.

Two years later, Laura started at another school. It took little more than a month for her teacher in the new school to recognise a learning difficulty and get in touch with Laura's parents. Jo and Maria were not surprised to find out that Laura had dyslexia but couldn't help asking themselves, 'Why my child?' Once the diagnosis was completed, the new school was very supportive and Jo and Maria relaxed as they learned more about it and learned to accept and understand it.

Maria observes that it was more difficult for them to find out than for their daughter, probably because adults have a much greater awareness of the problems that might lie in wait for their child. She recommends accepting and supporting your child, but also being accepting of yourself and acknowledging your hopes and fears. She suggests it pays to stay focused in the here and now rather than dwelling on problems in the future that may never even occur.

The hardest part for Jo and Maria was explaining to Laura that she was no different from other children, even though she had to work much harder than others to learn the same things.

She wishes she had found out sooner about the dyslexia and feels remorseful that she did not force the issue earlier and allowed Laura's first teacher to make her feel like a 'pushy parent'.

'I wish I had found out sooner that Laura had dyslexia.'

As Laura accepts her condition, she works hard at her schoolwork but is constantly tired.

Questions parents will have

As parents, you know your children better than anyone else. You have watched and observed their growth and development from birth. You see them in circumstances that may not be representative of how they behave in the classroom, especially if going to school is a new experience for them. Have confidence in your own observations of your child. If you sense something is wrong, it is worth looking into. And what if you are wrong? Much better that way round, than the other. The earlier you can recognise or diagnose dyslexia, the easier it will be to deal with. If left to linger undetected, it will slowly erode your child's self-esteem until it becomes a much bigger problem.

Finding out that your child is 'not like all the others' is a worrying prospect. I'm sure, as you read these parents' stories, they resonated with your own feelings of: Why me? Why my child? What long-term impact will this have on my child's self-esteem? What about my child's career? Is my child going to live a productive and happy life?

For the first few days or weeks following diagnosis, it will be as if someone has given you special glasses with highly focused lenses as you notice every little detail of daily life that depends on our ability to hold information in short-term memory, read instructions, follow directions, get from a to b and add things up. Organisation is critical to all levels of success in life, like remembering to pay your bills, taking medication, or picking up shopping on your way home from work. Frequently forgetting things is not conducive to an easy-going lifestyle.

Every little thing you are doing to help them right now is setting them up for success

As conscientious parents, one of our primary objectives is to raise our children to be independent and fully functioning in society. When we come home after a long day at work, and are up half the night comforting a child in tears over an upcoming spelling test, suddenly we start to wonder if they will ever be able to function without our help.

Don't worry. They will. And every little thing you are doing to help them right now is setting them up for the success you so desperately hope they will achieve. So take heart.

Take a little time to get used to the idea but, above all, take the advice of parents who have gone through this before. Find out all you can about your child's dyslexia and how to help overcome the obstacles. Share knowledge with other parents and support one another, and foster a good partnership with the school.

Read your child's educational assessment report until you know it by heart and understand it. Have your child re-assessed as he progresses through the educational system to ensure that progress is being made and is in line with your child's development. I provide many suggestions and solutions throughout the book, and there is a table of **Challenges and Solutions in the Classroom** that you will find helpful.

Take heart from the fact that your child will exhibit various exciting and interesting strengths and talents. Encourage your child with smiles and positivism to explore all his talents and not dwell on his shortcomings. Your child may not be destined to become a Leonardo da Vinci, an Einstein or a Walt Disney, but he may become successful and fulfilled in what he loves doing.

Chapter 3
Children's stories

My high school teachers would not have
believed I could have read all those briefs.
Early on I was told I probably wouldn't make it
through college. I knew I wasn't stupid, but I
had great hardships in school — since
second grade. Never give up hope. Take a
step back, because you can't learn anything
under pressure. And don't worry about the
label!

Erin Brockovich, environmental activist[6]

One of the greatest things about children is that they can
be surprisingly accepting of things that happen in their
lives, as long as they have the right level of support and care at
home and strategies for coping. I have seen children deal with
great misfortune and illnesses and, for the most part, I believe
children are incredibly resilient. At the same time, they are very
vulnerable and, without the appropriate framework of support
and nurturing, they can go through very tough times and, in the
worst case, turn out badly.

Children need coping strategies

It can be scary for children to find out something is 'wrong'
with them.

The parents whose stories I shared with you chose not to
look at their children in that way and are raising them with
great optimism. You will see how positively their attitudes have
reflected in the attitudes of their children.

Children's stories

Sally

Sally now has nine GCSEs, seven of which are 'A' grades. Not bad for someone diagnosed with a learning disability when she was nine years old! Sally's achievements are living proof a child with dyslexia can excel in school even if the diagnosis is not accomplished when first entering the school system.

Sally's assessment and subsequent diagnosis with dyslexia were prompted by the fact that she didn't always understand what she was reading, and she had difficulty getting ideas down on paper.

As she progressed through school, she says she had a lot of trouble finishing things on time, especially exams. She became frustrated trying to meet the deadlines that were set for assignments. She also had trouble retaining a long list of items when given to her in one go. Spelling and grammar were always difficult too. Maths and English were the subjects she least enjoyed:

> 'I felt I was not very good at Maths and English and struggled to understand some concepts that others seemed to find easy.'

She found it especially disheartening in English when her essays would be returned covered in corrections even though she worked really hard on them, and excelled at planning the essay content. She describes her frustration with an essay assignment about a Shakespeare play:

> 'I knew what I had to write, but I couldn't seem to get it on paper in the way I wanted. I must have written about 10 drafts of it, each time having to get someone to read it before I felt it was okay.'

Outside school, Sally remembers spending a lot longer than the other kids on her homework. She also had to write things down in order to remember everything she had to accomplish that day.

Despite her dyslexia, she was always really good at managing her time, planning (not writing) essays and she became good at reading. Her favourite subjects are food technology and the sciences – she especially loves experiencing the hands-on element of doing lab experiments and being creative with food. She wants to go to university to study nutrition.

Although she has overcome her dyslexia to a large degree and has excelled academically in spite of it, she still finds it frustrating when she struggles with something with which other people probably don't have a problem. She is grateful to her parents for patiently reading through her work and working with her in the areas where she needed help.

Jay

Jay, aged twelve, remembers finding things difficult as far back as age three, when he was at playgroup. He found out about his dyslexia when he turned seven years old. He says the things he has the most trouble with are reading and spelling. Mum says he also lacks confidence in himself. When I asked Jay how he felt about having dyslexia, he admitted that it made him feel stupid at first but, now that he is learning to understand it, he feels better about it.

Jay is great at making things, being creative, constructing things and drawing. His favourite subject at school is art and the subjects he dislikes the most are maths and English. Jay feels very supported by his mum and dad, who have arranged extra lessons for him in school, practise his reading skills at home and support him with his homework.

Jack

Although Jack describes himself as 'grumpy', when you meet him, you can't help but notice that he has an easy-going, charming personality. Jack loves sport and excels at swimming. He also loves history. Now 14 years old, he remembers having trouble in school from the very beginning and was diagnosed with dyslexia at the age of seven.

His most hated subject is English, especially writing sentences that make sense, spelling and punctuation, and he consequently has difficulty writing long stories (which is also quite typical of plenty of people who do not have dyslexia) and doing comprehensions.

Jack told me that having dyslexia made it hard for him to keep up with others in class and he often felt that he needed more explanation than the teacher gave during a lesson. When I asked him what was the best thing his parents have done for him he said:

> 'My parents have helped me believe that I'm good enough for anything.'

Laura

Laura cannot remember a time when she did not have trouble with schoolwork. Early on she had trouble memorising the way words were spelled as well as her times tables. As she got older, she had trouble understanding things and was unable to analyse books the way other students could. She also had a lot of trouble revising for tests and exams.

Laura was diagnosed with dyslexia when she was seven years old. One thing she struggled with a lot was remembering instructions from her teachers. She needed things to be written down or repeated very slowly one at a time so she could remember them. She always felt that she missed the most obvious answer that others came up with and found that her mind had taken the long way round, producing a time-consuming or an obscure answer.

On the other hand, Laura is quick to recognise patterns and, even though her long way round of thinking failed to produce the obvious answer, she often came up with a creative, out-of-the-box, answer.

Her favourite subjects at school were history and geography and the subjects she hated the most were science, maths and languages. She found science boring and incredibly hard work, and had trouble grasping the concepts and scientific explanations. She described maths as boring and uninteresting, and she experienced a lot of difficulty in French and Spanish because she had trouble memorising the sentence structures and verb endings.

When I asked Laura how she feels about having dyslexia, she said simply:

> 'It's something I have, and I have learned coping strategies.'

In spite of her dyslexia, Laura is now happily studying at university.

Questions children will have

My sample students come from homes where parents had their children assessed and diagnosis was made early enough to make a difference in the child's academic career. Children nonetheless have questions. The hardest question to answer is, 'Why me?'

Diagnosis was made early enough to make a difference in the child's academic career

The simplest way to deal with this question is to explain that we are all different. Some of us are good athletes, others can sing. Some have blond hair and blue eyes and others have black hair and brown eyes. We might be dark-skinned, light-skinned, and all shades in between. It's the same thing with the way our brains work. Some of us think linearly and others think non-linearly. It's just what we've got. And we're all blessed with gifts and talents.

Other questions your child might have will be practical, such as 'Can you help me with my homework?' You might have to deal with issues of frustration such as 'How come I can never remember to bring my swimsuit to school on Mondays?' The easiest way to deal with frustrating issues like forgetting to take things to school is to use a calendar or chart posted where the child can easily check it every day on the way out. Charts for organisation, homework and revision are life-savers for children with learning difficulties, and I have included some charts at the back of this book.

Dyslexic learners often feel frustrated and misunderstood. Sources of exasperation for many children at school are the negative comments made by their teachers, such as 'You could have put more effort into your homework' or 'Messy handwriting' or 'Too many errors, please resubmit'. Teachers who are aware of dyslexia and other learning difficulties can find out the exact extent of children's problems by reading their specialist teacher assessment or educational psychologist's report. It's also a good idea for teachers to find out just how much time and effort is being put into children's homework so that unreasonable demands or negative comments aren't made, as these can have a lasting, detrimental effect on children's self-esteem.

If your child is attending learning support classes for his dyslexia or specific learning difference and has to leave his regular lesson at set times, he will probably have questions about why he is being singled out. The chances are he won't be the only one receiving learning support classes, which is a comfort to many children. Parents need to explain that it will be for a relatively short time to give children a boost so that certain aspects of learning become easier. Often children grow to love the individual attention, which actually builds, rather than undermines, their ability and self-confidence. The learning support teacher can be a source of comfort, where children can vent their upset and frustration and can feel that someone is on their side and is completely supporting them.

Focus on the positive skills your child has

If you focus on the positive skills your child has, it is easier for him to accept that there are some things he finds tricky.

PART TWO
Understanding Dyslexia and Learning Difficulties

Chapter 4
What is dyslexia?

Dyslexia can slow you down but not stop you
from your goals. Understanding what it is can
be most enlightening.

Michael Charles Messineo, author[7]

Even though dyslexia is such a common 'condition', some
people may be unaware that it is recognised in the UK
under the Equality Act (2010, previously known as the Disability
Discrimination Act 1995 (DDA)) and is considered to be a
disability. In the UK, employers have a responsibility under the
Equality Act to make 'reasonable adjustments' for employees
with dyslexia.

In the UK, schools have a responsibility to comply with the
Equality Act and the Special Educational Needs and Disability
Act 2001 (SENDA). In the USA, the relevant Acts are the
Individuals with Disabilities Education Act (IDEA 2004) and the
Rehabilitation Act (1973) section 504 and, in Australia, the
Disability Discrimination Act.

The terms used for dyslexia vary across the world from
Special Educational Needs and Disability (SEND) in the UK to
Learning Disability (LD) in Canada and the US, and Learning
Difficulty or Learning Disorder in Australia and New Zealand, all
of which treat dyslexia as a disability.

Estimates of people with dyslexia from English-speaking
countries vary between 10% and 20% of the population
depending on the country, the government, the way statistics
are gathered and the reality in our schools. In the US, the
Society for Neuroscience suggests that as many as 43.5 million
Americans may have dyslexia.[8]

Even at a conservative figure of 10% of the population, we are still talking about 30 million people in the US, 6 million in the UK, 5 million in South Africa, 3 million in Canada and 3 million in New Zealand and Australia together.

Educationalists should view dyslexia as a learning ability rather than a learning disability

In the UK, dyslexia is often used as an umbrella term for Specific Learning Difficulties (SpLD), a term that covers a wide variety of 'difficulties'. Many people use this term synonymously with dyslexia, but it is now generally accepted that dyslexia is only one of a group of difficulties.

As a person who has dyslexia, I dislike the word 'difficulties' as it has the negative implication of a 'problem'. Perhaps we could use the word 'style' – 'Individual Learning Style'? I believe that people with dyslexia have a unique collection of learning styles and qualities that should be identified so that they can achieve their potential at school and in the workplace. In the classroom, dyslexia has its own unique collection of learning challenges, particularly if teachers deliver in a left-brain style. I believe educationalists should view dyslexia as a learning ability rather than a learning disability.

Dyslexia definitions

Most research suggests that dyslexia is *not* a result of low intelligence, nor is it based on ethnic origin or class. It is not a middle class excuse for underachievement at school. It is not just about difficulties with reading, speaking, spelling, listening and writing; and it is not because of poor eyesight or hearing. There are, however, medical conditions that can sometimes cause similar symptoms to dyslexia. Poor eyesight can cause difficulties reading and learning how to read; poor hearing can cause misunderstanding and speech and language problems and can lead to an inability to learn as quickly as others.

If you suspect that your child has dyslexia, but you are not sure, certainly arrange for vision and hearing tests to rule out the possibility of any physical problems.

So what is dyslexia? I have chosen two definitions, one British and one American. The British Dyslexia Association defines dyslexia as:

> ... a specific learning difficulty which mainly affects the development of literacy and language related skills.
>
> It is likely to be present at birth and to be lifelong in its effects.
>
> It is characterised by difficulties with phonological processing, rapid naming, working memory, processing speed, and the automatic development of skills that may not match up to an individual's other cognitive abilities.
>
> It tends to be resistant to conventional teaching methods, but its effects can be mitigated by appropriate[ly] specific intervention, including the application of information technology and supportive counselling.[9]

The 'conventional teaching methods' mentioned by the BDA were traditionally delivered using left-brain teaching methods. Most children find left-brain learning boring and uninspiring. Teaching is most effective when it matches the children's learning preferences.

Researchers and educators are constantly proving that, by adapting the way we teach, using fun, multisensory (a mixture of visual, auditory and kinaesthetic) teaching methods and addressing the individual learning styles (preferences) and Multiple Intelligences of children who have dyslexia, we can reach and engage dyslexic and non-dyslexic learners more effectively at the same time.

What's more, we can provide children with strategies and tools for learning that make it much easier for them than using conventional teaching methods. By adapting the way we teach, using multisensory teaching methods, all learners can be reached more effectively.

The International Dyslexia Association[10] defines dyslexia as:

> ... a language-based learning disability. Dyslexia refers
> to a cluster of symptoms, which result in people having
> difficulties with specific language skills, particularly
> reading. Students with dyslexia usually experience
> difficulties with other language skills such as spelling,
> writing, and pronouncing words. Dyslexia affects
> individuals throughout their lives; however, its impact
> can change at different stages in a person's life. It is
> referred to as a learning disability because dyslexia can
> make it very difficult for a student to succeed
> academically in the typical instructional environment,
> and in its more severe forms, will qualify a student for
> special education, special accommodations, or extra
> support services.

Many studies have been conducted on the brains of
children and adults with dyslexia. There is overwhelming
consensus among scientists that the left temporal regions of the
brain are not sufficiently active in people with dyslexia, proving
that there is a physical correlation between learning disabilities
and the physical make-up of the brain.

Typically, the areas of the brain that support both visualisation
and language are affected, supporting the theory dyslexic
difficulties are the result of a combination of phonological, visual
processing and auditory processing differences.

Dyslexia is a blanket term for a variety of possible
characteristics associated with a neurological condition that
makes the brain function in a different way from the brain of
individuals who do not have dyslexia. There are several other
'conditions' that may have some similar and overlapping
symptoms to dyslexia. Consequently, dyslexia is hard to identify
without a formal diagnosis.

These other 'conditions' include dyspraxia, dyscalculia,
dysgraphia and dysnomia (among others). Other 'disorders'
within the term 'Specific Learning Difficulties' include: Auditory
Processing Disorder, Visual Processing Disorder, Sensory
Processing Disorder, Attention Deficit Disorder or Attention
Deficit Hyperactivity Disorder (ADD or ADHD), and Autistic

Spectrum Disorder (including Asperger Syndrome). These are all described in more detail in the following chapters.

People with dyslexia are often highly intuitive, insightful, creative, musical, sporty and intelligent

In general, if you suspect that any of these 'conditions' is present in your child, I would recommend a complete assessment by an educational psychologist or specialist teacher. An assessment will measure your child's cognitive skills, academic potential, strengths and weaknesses on multiple levels, and a detailed report will be produced, so that you know exactly where your child's strengths and challenges lie. You will then be better equipped to deal with the situation and learn what tools and techniques you need to give your child to arm him in an academic environment that is geared towards non-dyslexic learners – although this is gradually changing. The identification and assessment process is so important that I devote a whole chapter to it: **The benefit of having an educational assessment**.

Although this book deals primarily with dyslexia, I do address dyspraxia, dyscalculia and dysgraphia in several areas. You need to research the specific 'condition' that applies to your child and be guided by the recommendations in the assessment report. No matter which 'condition' is dominant, you will need much love and patience to help your child cope. Once you have this information (and support), it becomes much easier both for you and your child to manage.

If your child suffers from any of these 'dys' 'conditions', you will also discover *wonderful* characteristics that might be a direct result of your child thinking a little differently, a little more creatively and a little out of the box. People with dyslexia are often highly intuitive, insightful, creative, musical, sporty and intelligent. They often have special talents that are bursting to be acknowledged.

Many positive characteristics can result from dyslexia, to the extent that it has often been called a gift rather than a disability, but in my experience, many dyslexic learners do not see it as a gift, as they battle their way to read, write, spell and remember information. Their frequent tears are evidence of how unhappy they feel without the right level of support, which is why it is *vital* to help your child focus on his strengths.

Characteristics of dyslexia

The following table gives general characteristics that may be present in varying degrees in an individual with dyslexia. Individuals will not manifest every one of these characteristics. For example, some dyslexic learners may not have a problem with directions or time. Others may not have difficulties with organisational skills. Each child is different, although there tends to be a common pattern or thread. You can also refer to indicators of dyslexia by age from the British Dyslexia Association in the **Appendix**.

Mild, moderate and severe dyslexia

The determination of dyslexia is based upon a formal diagnostic assessment involving several different tests of ability and attainment. Most assessments give reading, spelling, writing and numeracy ability in standardised scores, percentiles and, sometimes, age (years and months), that is, exactly what age the child is performing at.

Many parents find comparing their child's ability in years and months a much easier comparison than interpreting standardised scores. However, the degree of severity does not line up exactly against age comparisons. A two-year difference at a young age can indicate more severe dyslexia than the same difference at a later age. For example, a child who is ten, but performing at the level of an eight-year-old, indicates a higher degree of difficulty than a sixteen-year-old performing at the level of a fourteen-year-old, so standardised scores and percentiles are better comparisons.

In the UK, It is estimated that at least 6% of children have mild to moderate dyslexia, with 4% having severe dyslexia. In severe cases, some children may still struggle at mainstream school despite having one-to-one intervention. In such cases, many parents choose to send their child to a specialist dyslexia school.

General Characteristics of Dyslexia

- Confusion between letters and words such as: 'b' and 'd'; 'p' and 'q'; 'th', 'f' and 'v'; 'was' and 'saw'; 'on' and 'no'; 'left' and 'felt'
- Difficulty reading and recognising letter patterns
- Problems understanding what is read
- Difficulty spelling (relating to letter pattern recognition)
- Difficulty processing sounds
- Mispronouncing words or speaking words in the wrong order
- Problems processing language
- Struggling to learn how to tell the time
- Difficulty remembering times tables
- Difficulty remembering formulae or performing wordy maths questions
- Sequencing: difficulty organising or processing information sequentially
- Difficulty with hand-to-eye coordination (a little clumsy; trips over a lot; bumps into things; difficulty catching/throwing a ball or hopping)
- Difficulty planning stories or essays
- Difficulty remembering homework, names, places, directions
- Difficulty multi-tasking
- Difficulty getting dressed (doing up zips; putting shoes on the wrong foot)
- Overwhelmed by too many instructions at once and difficulty remembering/processing lists of instructions or information
- Difficulty with directions; may lose their way even on familiar routes

- Mixing up right/left, north/south, up/down etc.
- Organisational problems with day-to-day tasks
- Time management problems; trouble conceptualising time and may frequently be late, miss appointments or not accomplish tasks within a given time
- Poor concentration; short attention span
- Poor short-term memory, often coupled with very good long-term memory
- Processing problems: visual or auditory (not seeing and hearing)
- Easily distracted, restless or with behavioural problems resulting from frustration at sitting still and being made to read/write/listen etc.
- Tendency to 'right-brain thinking'

Recognising dyslexia at different ages

In most cases, the symptoms of dyslexia are more noticeable when children are at the age when they should be making progress in reading and writing, and yet begin to underperform in the classroom, generally from about seven years old. In my family, I knew my children had some form of learning challenge around the age of four to five years, and I am able to detect the possibility of learning difficulties in most pupils from around five years, but I advise testing after seven years of age.

Today, testing is more prevalent in schools than previously, so it is possible some older children or adults who have dyslexia have never been diagnosed, or were diagnosed at a late age.

You may even remember problems you had at school, because you can see similar patterns in your child. Several parents say that they have always known their child had some sort of learning difficulty prior to a diagnosis of dyslexia. In my experience, parents are the experts in knowing if there is a problem, unless they are in denial.

Younger children

Late talking can be indicative of many different things but is not necessarily a sign of dyslexia. If your child was a late talker, do not assume that anything is wrong. However, taken in combination with other symptoms, you may get a sense that something is amiss. Other indications in children can be lateness in learning to walk, or skipping the crawling stage, instead shuffling around on their bottoms or tummies and then going straight to walking. When learning to dress themselves, they may persistently put their shoes on the wrong feet long after other kids have mastered left and right shoes. They may have trouble distinguishing words and concepts like 'left', 'right', 'up' and 'down', or remembering rhyming words in nursery rhymes. Dyslexic learners often mix up words by substituting similar-sounding ones that have a different meaning, such as 'fireplace' instead of 'fireworks'.

Another common symptom in young children with dyslexia is mispronouncing certain words and switching the first letters of a word pair (known as spoonerisms). Examples are:

'par cark'	for 'car park'
'belly jeans'	for 'jelly beans'

They may also be slower at learning new words, learning to write their name or have trouble remembering nursery rhymes, colours, shapes and so on. You may notice that they are slower to develop fine motor skills such as holding a crayon or pencil correctly or colouring between the lines. There is often a wide range of 'normal' among siblings being raised together, and not all children learn to do things at the 'right' or same time. The best guide, if your child is still young, is your own intuition.

By the time children reach primary school, it becomes easier to recognise learning difficulties. A child who is having a lot of trouble with reading or writing, or who once loved to read and develops a dislike for it, may be presenting characteristics of dyslexia. A primary-school-aged child with dyslexia may also mix up certain letters or misread common words. You may also notice that he is beginning to recite from memory rather than reading each word.

It is possible to have younger children assessed but it is better to wait until they are over seven to gain a more holistic and comprehensive assessment.

Older children

Pre-adolescent children may experience more than normal difficulties with reading and writing, and procrastinate when it is time for homework or revision.

They may invent excuses for forgetting to hand homework in and take steps to avoid being called on to read aloud in class or similar situations. You, or their teacher, may notice that they are not 'getting' spelling strategies, or perhaps they remember spellings for a test but frequently spell the same word incorrectly in essays, or they cannot recognise common words. They may have inconsistent or unclear handwriting. You may notice that they are having trouble remembering things, such as bringing the right equipment to and from school. Their behaviour may be poor, and they may not be feeling good about themselves.

**They remember spellings for a test,
but frequently spell the same word
incorrectly in free writing**

Adults

Adults with dyslexia often try to hide their difficulties by avoiding situations where they have to read aloud, write, complete forms or analyse written information, although they may be very articulate in spoken language.

They often depend on remembering facts rather than reading, and may rely on others to take notes or prefer not to write reports or emails. They may be intuitive and have good people skills; they may also have excellent thinking skills and work in jobs that require a high degree of creativity, such as design, engineering or marketing. Sometimes, they are in jobs that are beneath their intellectual capability because they have avoided situations or careers where they would need to do a lot of reading or writing.

Phonemic awareness and dyslexia

Phonemic awareness is the ability to recognise sounds in words and is an important part of being able to read (and spell). It is also considered an important element in the ability to listen and to function intelligently. People with poor phonemic awareness may have difficulty reading, writing, listening or speaking.

People with reading difficulties, such as dyslexia, have repeatedly proved to have poor phonemic awareness

When you start learning to read, you are taught to sound out words such as c-a-t and d-o-g. With poor phonemic awareness, it is difficult to identify the individual letter sounds or syllables that make up a word. Thus, it is hard to comprehend that c-a-t and c-o-t have the same starting and ending letters. The word 'cat' is made up of the sounds 'c', 'a' and 't' – so it has three sounds but only one syllable. People with poor phonemic awareness have trouble identifying how many sounds are in a single word. They may have trouble blending sounds (e.g. 't' and 'h' to make 'th' as in **the, th**ink, **th**ought or 'o' and 'a' to make 'oa' as in b**oa**t), or associating words that rhyme, like 'pear' and 'hair'.

It's easy to understand having poor phonemic awareness makes it difficult to learn how to read. People with reading difficulties such as dyslexia have repeatedly proven to have poor phonemic awareness.

Although some children manage to memorise whole words and shapes of words and seem to have less difficulty reading, there comes a time when the lack of phonemic awareness manifests itself when they are trying to sound out (decode) longer words or spell words (encode).

Reading is one of the major ways of building vocabulary and developing intuitive grammar skills and an intelligent grasp of language. It is also one of the primary ways in which we acquire knowledge of our world and subjects that matter to us.

When deprived of the ability to read, we risk being considered less intelligent, less knowledgeable and less articulate than our peers. Since reading begins at an early age, poor readers often have a weak foundation on which to start building their knowledge of the world. When the foundation is weak, the structure quickly crumbles.

Individuals have differing amounts of skills and talents. Lacking a skill does not mean we cannot be taught, using carefully directed methods to acquire it. Once the problem has been identified, we can explore the many programmes to teach phonemic awareness skills and phonics.

Difficulties with reading

Reading can be one of the most frustrating tasks for people with dyslexia, especially since almost everything in the academic and working environment depends on reading successfully. Manifestation of short-term memory or speed of processing problems, in combination with some of the other difficulties associated with dyslexia, brings with it a variety of difficulties that might present themselves while reading.

Reading Difficulties
• Reading slowly
• Reading with hesitation
• Feeling very tired after reading
• Finding it hard to focus on reading for very long
• Frequently forgetting the meaning of unfamiliar words even after they have been explained
• Trouble sounding out unfamiliar words
• Not comprehending what is being read, because effort is being focused on decoding individual words
• Difficulty remembering what has just been read, or processing the information contained in the text
• Needing to read something more than once to make sense of it
• Not noticing certain words or mixing up the order of words such that it changes the meaning of the sentence
• Omitting small words: the, a, of

- Frequently losing one's place while reading
- Difficulty reading black print on bright white paper
- Letters or words 'moving' on the page
- Suffering from eye strain and/or headaches

If your child has been diagnosed with a specific learning difficulty, taking written exams may be a problem. Exam papers need to be read carefully in order to answer the questions correctly. If your child has a tendency to miss out small words when reading or is unable to pronounce a word, this can have a significant impact on understanding exam questions.

Under certain circumstances, he may qualify for special conditions at exam time, usually in the form of additional time, and in some cases, a reader or a scribe may be recommended. This can be the case at all stages of education: primary, secondary and university.

Difficulties with writing (getting ideas down)

The skills of reading and writing fluency (not handwriting) are closely related. A child who reads often and well is more likely to understand the skills required for proficient writing, such as having good ideas, story plots, sequencing events and a wide range of exciting vocabulary.

A child who has difficulty reading and reads infrequently is less likely to develop proficient writing skills than a child who is an avid reader. Furthermore, the characteristics of dyslexia bring challenges to writing, as they do to reading. These may be due to attention, language difficulties, short-term memory, processing speed, sequencing, planning, higher order thinking or motor skills, for example.

Handwriting difficulties are a separate issue and are discussed under the sections **Characteristics of Dyspraxia and Dysgraphia**. A summary of writing difficulties that might be present is in the following table.

Writing Difficulties

- Inability to start because they panic or can't think of a good story line
- Can't put great ideas down on paper because of sequencing or organisational problems
- Frustrated at being unable to express themselves clearly in writing
- Writing slowly with many revisions. Inability to understand or reorganise their thought process when they read back what they have written
- Missing out words, or mixing up the word order or tenses
- Misspelling words, with a particular tendency to spell phonetically or use only words they can spell, thereby limiting vocabulary
- Writing too fast in order to capture thoughts before they forget them (because they are not using a story plan)

Memory and dyslexia

The phenomenon of a poor short-term memory can be pronounced in people who have dyslexia, dyscalculia, dyspraxia and other specific learning difficulties. Memory is made up of several parts, including sensory memory, which is very fleeting, short-term memory, where we process sensory inputs and determine whether to remember them or not, and long-term memory, where we are able to store information for a lifetime.

Good short-term memory is fundamental to absorbing information and learning it. It is also a vital part of the brain's processing system when we analyse information to solve problems, because it is essentially where long-term information is brought for short-term thinking and problem solving (working memory). When the short-term memory is weak or impaired, the act of learning becomes extremely difficult.

Many parents are confused by the possibility of their child having short-term memory problems when he seems to have a great long-term memory for general knowledge or experiences. The **Memory and Memory Strategies** chapter covers this topic in greater detail.

Positive qualities of dyslexia

Teachers, educators and child psychologists are beginning to understand that it is no longer sufficient to measure a child's intelligence or performance in school solely in terms of traditional reading, writing, spelling and mathematics skills.

Dyslexic learners exhibit many positive qualities, especially in areas of creativity and big vision thinking. Some famous people with dyslexia are credited with making leaps in human understanding enabling the human race to make progress in important ways, particularly in science, maths and inventions.

However, while you can measure a child's ability in maths by administering a test with questions that have specific answers, it is much harder to measure an individual's 'creativity quotient' or 'emotional intelligence'. For this reason, a child's special skills may not be recognised in the normal run of tests administered by schools.

Below is a list of positive qualities dyslexic learners may exhibit as a result of their constant battle to overcome learning difficulties. These are not necessarily acknowledged 'traits' of dyslexia but, because they have to work much harder than other children, those with dyslexia often learn to be:

- Inspiring
- Resilient
- Determined
- Strong-minded
- Hard-working
- Persistent
- Resourceful
- Inventive
- Motivated
- Lateral thinker

Despite the fact that dyslexic learners may not initially exhibit strengths in the areas of reading and writing, many go on to do outstanding work in professions where these skills are important to success, such as politics, law, business, teaching, writing, acting, science and design.

The key to dealing with dyslexia is learning to leverage your positive skills, while minimising your weaker skills by implementing coping strategies. A dyslexic learner who is aware of his learning difficulties and is well equipped with coping strategies can be a powerful force in his own life and the lives of others.

People with dyslexia can become people who make a big difference and further progress in the world in a multitude of small ways, and sometimes in much bigger ways.

Positive Qualities of Having Dyslexia

- Ability to think in pictures and images
- Ability to make connections between seemingly unrelated things (resulting in some of the creative theories in science that have subsequently proven to be true)
- Being innovative
- Being insightful and intuitive
- Big vision, big picture thinking
- Creativity
- Good imagination
- Good general knowledge
- Articulate and good at creative or writing poetry
- Empathic
- Energetic
- Focused
- Good intra-personal skills
- Good verbal skills
- Good visual-spatial skills and three-dimensional thinking
- High emotional intelligence
- Lateral thinking and good problem-solving skills
- Out-of-the-box thinking
- Talents, such as: music, art, sports, drama, dance, cookery, science, 3D design, architecture, technology, entrepreneurial skills, among many others

---

Famous people with dyslexia

There have been many famous people throughout history who have or had dyslexia and dyslexia is present in several royal families.

Dyslexic thinkers have been responsible for some of the biggest strides in human evolution. Without their extraordinary thinking ability and out-of-the box ideas, we might still be struggling with ideas such as human evolution and how to put satellites in space.

Ronald D. Davis, in his book *The Gift of Dyslexia*, recounts a time when he appeared on a television show, talked about his dyslexia and listed several famous people who have dyslexia. The show hostess commented on how amazing it was that so many people could be geniuses in spite of having dyslexia. Ron comments she missed the point entirely: they were famous because of, not in spite of, their dyslexia. He goes on to say:[11]

> Having dyslexia won't make every dyslexic a genius, but it is good for the self-esteem of all dyslexics to know their minds work in exactly the same way as the minds of great geniuses. It is also important for them to know that having a problem with reading, writing, spelling or maths doesn't mean they are dumb or stupid. The same mental function that produces a genius can also produce those problems.

While it is encouraging for you as parents to know that your child has the potential to follow in the footsteps of some of the most extraordinary people in history, we need to be careful not to put pressure on a young child already wrestling with being unable to do some of the things that look so easy to his peers, by holding up to him an Albert Einstein or a Charles Darwin.

The key to their success has been doing what they love and what they are good at

However, to get an idea of the many different professions of successful people with dyslexia, take a look at the list I have composed of famous and infamous people with dyslexia on my website, **www.carolinafrohlich.co.uk**. They are from all walks of life and have clearly made their mark on the world. It is incredible to see how many famous people have dyslexia. Their accomplishments have been despite, or because of, having dyslexia. The key to their success has been perseverance and determination, and *doing what they love and what they are good at.*

Chapter 5
What causes dyslexia?

Three-dimensional thinking was what was created by the dyslexia problem. I could design these things in my head.

Bennett Strahan, architect[12]

Experts suggest there are many possible risk factors that cause dyslexia, which range from biological (genetic and neurological), motor control and cognitive factors (phonological deficit, processing, developmental delay) to behavioural or even environmental influences (school, home or literacy environment). While it remains unclear what exactly causes dyslexia, there is more evidence to support the view that, because dyslexia runs strongly in families, there is a genetic link. In my family, my children are blessed with having a mum with dyslexia.

Developmental and acquired dyslexia

There are generally considered to be two types of dyslexia, 'developmental' and 'acquired'. Developmental dyslexia is often hereditary. You may or may not recognise the hereditary chain it has followed in your family, since it was recognised far less in earlier generations than currently and may not have been diagnosed.

Much research suggests that it is a neurological condition, which means it is caused by physical differences in the brain and is not induced or caused by anything external. You cannot cause your child to have developmental dyslexia by being a neglectful parent! People are born with it, and there is no known physical 'correction' available for it.

The genetics links to understanding developmental dyslexia are complex and scientists are continually undergoing studies to link dyslexia to genetic factors and chromosomes. Recent research about genes on chromosomes 1, 2, 3, 6, 15, 18 in the human genome[13] has suggested links to dyslexia; and a study conducted in the UK suggests there is 'strong evidence that KIAA0319 on chromosome 6p is a susceptibility gene for developmental dyslexia'.[14]

Other studies suggest that 'the combination of genetic and functional imaging data show a link between genes and brain functioning during reading tasks in subjects with RD (reading disability)'.[15]

The Dyslexia Research Trust reports that 'KIAA0319 has turned out to be involved with controlling the early development of the brain. It may also underlie the unfortunate tendency of the immune system of dyslexics to cause allergies, eczema etc.'[16]

You may be interested in a major research project called 'The project NEURODYS', undertaken by the European Commission's Sixth Framework Programme 'to clarify the biological bases of developmental dyslexia',[17] and to confirm relations between dyslexia, genes and brain regions.

Acquired dyslexia differs from developmental dyslexia in that children are not born with it, but may 'acquire' it, possibly due to suffering frequent colds, sore throats or early ear infections known as 'glue ear' (otitis media), or conductive hearing loss. It is likely that the ears become blocked, which causes loss of hearing in the early years of a child's life. Some children may need grommets inserted into the eardrum in order to improve their hearing. If the difficulty is not picked up at an early stage, the developing brain does not make links between the sounds it hears, which possibly results in a delay in acquiring phonemic awareness.

Left-brain, right-brain dominance

Roger W Sperry, Nobel Prize winner, discovered the concept of two brains and left-brain right-brain theory. While left-brain, right-brain theory is often over-generalised, and labels such as 'logical' or 'creative' have been linked to left and right laterals of the brain, these labels need to be treated carefully. Although a lateral dominance is measurable, many of these characteristics exist in both sides.

The human brain is divided into the left and right hemispheres. Researchers have found that the right hemisphere of the dyslexic learner's brain is larger than that of non-dyslexic learners. We believe this is why people with dyslexia tend to be right-brain dominant, meaning that they are often gifted in areas that are typically associated with right-brain creative functions such as art, music, spatial skills, colour, images, 3-D visualisation, people skills, expressing emotions and intuition. The left hemisphere of the brain is associated with logical, analytical, critical thinking, mathematical, reasoning, language, writing and scientific skills.

Whether your child seems to be left-brained, right-brained or a balance of both does not indicate whether or not he is intelligent, but rather what his personal style is like, including his learning preference, personality and natural gifts. Typically, academic subjects are more easily mastered by those who appear to be left-brain dominant. Teaching of academic subjects is often directed at left-brain thinking, which is analytical and logical rather than creative and artistic.

Teachers and lecturers use a variety of techniques focused on listening and reading, such as oral presentations, stand-up lectures and written hand-outs and, in the past, made less use of techniques such as hands-on experimentation, visual aids, colour coding, charts, diagrams, role play, acting and field work.

Left-brained or whole-brained thinkers might not experience difficulty with these traditional methods of teaching, whereas right-brained thinkers will constantly be called on to exercise the part of their brain that is their less natural inclination.

With reading, we know from fMRI scans (functional Magnetic Resonance Imaging) that activity levels in the left hemisphere of the brain (Broca's area, Wernicke's area pariotemporal and occiptotemporal regions) are lower and function inefficiently in people with dyslexia. Broca's area is responsible for the production of speech; Wernicke's area is important for language development and the comprehension of speech. The synaptic paths active in the brain of people with dyslexia differ from those of non-dyslexic readers, meaning that the dyslexic brain functions in a different way from the non-dyslexic brain when performing reading tasks.

When children first learn to read, there is much activity in the right part of the brain. As non-dyslexic learners acquire reading skills, activity moves to the left side. In dyslexic learners, there continues to be more activity in the right side of the brain, indicating that the reading process in the dyslexic brain follows a different path. This may also explain why dyslexia is often not easily diagnosed until a child starts to develop reading skills.

Visual processing problems

In some people with dyslexia, visual paths in the brain are thought to be affected, as well as the cerebral cortex and the cerebellum. You may know that we see an image upside down until the brain corrects it for us and turns it the right way up. This processing takes a lot of brainpower. With visual processing problems, the eyes are not the main source of the problem, rather the way the brain perceives and interprets information sent through the eyes.

Many dyslexic readers report that words are blurry or appear to wobble, which makes it hard for them to keep focused on a page of writing. It also explains why some say they see letters move around, letter reversals, wavy lines or have trouble keeping their place while reading.

Some children experience sensitivity to light. For example, bright white paper with black writing can appear distorted and hard to read. This sensitivity to light, known as Irlen® Syndrome or Scotopic Sensitivity Syndrome, can be a part of the problem for children and adults who have eye problems, or symptoms of dyslexia, dyspraxia, ADHD, chronic fatigue syndrome, behaviour and emotional problems, migraine or headaches.

The Irlen® organisation in the UK provides this explanation:

> Having Irlen Syndrome prevents many people from reading effectively and efficiently. The problems are caused by the way in which the brain interprets the

visual information that is being sent through the eyes. Individuals with Irlen Syndrome perceive reading material and/or their environment differently. They must constantly make adaptations or compensate for their eye problems.[18]

John Stein of Magdalen College, Oxford, has studied the physical differences in the brains of learning 'disabled' individuals, including those with dyslexia.[19] His studies show that, in people with dyslexia, the visual path from the eyes to the brain is deficient. When you look at a word on a page, your eyes have to fixate on the word only momentarily in order to recognise it. However, that fixation requires your eyes to stabilise and be very still for a brief moment.

In people with dyslexia, it has been proven that the link between the retina and the visual processing system in the brain works inefficiently due to a physical difference in the brain's magnocellular (M-) cells. M-cells are neurons located within the magnocellular layer of the lateral geniculate nucleus. A weak magnocellular system causes unstable vision, and therefore difficulty fixating on words in order to read them properly.

If your child is complaining of having headaches, sore eyes or has difficulty reading, I suggest first having a routine eye test to rule out short- or long-sightedness and, if the symptoms persist, it is important to be checked out by a behavioural optometrist, or a certified Irlen diagnostician. Many times, children cannot tell you they have a visual problem, because they don't understand their symptoms or realise that they aren't seeing correctly.

If your child is diagnosed with Scotopic Sensitivity Syndrome or Irlen® Syndrome, he may be prescribed colour-tinted lenses or filters that reduce or eliminate the glare that causes some readers to experience perceptual difficulties. For other children who experience this difficulty, the solution might be as simple as using cream-coloured paper and dark blue print, or a plastic coloured overlay reading ruler to reduce glare.

Some children may be prescribed 'behavioural vision therapy' to improve eye movement control, eye focusing and coordination, and to manage peripheral vision, colour perception, gross and fine visual–motor, or visual perception.

The Irlen Institute and the College of Optometrists in Vision Development have a facility to search across the whole world for local test centres, or you can search for Behavioural Optometrists in the UK and Ireland.

For further information go to: **www.irlen.com**, **www.covd.org** and **www.babo.co.uk**.

Auditory processing problems

Another theory about the physical cause of dyslexia is an auditory processing weakness, which means that children do not easily process what is being said. Children may be able to repeat words back precisely but the meaning of the message is lost, not understood (not processed properly). Where auditory pathways are weak, some people with dyslexia also experience sensitivity to sound and background noise.

Hearing is one of the traditional senses and is the ability to perceive sound by detecting vibrations through the ear. The ear is a delicate and highly detailed sensory organ that is divided into the outer, middle and inner ear.

In order to hear, our ear must direct the sound waves into the hearing part of the inner ear, the cochlea, which senses the fluctuations in air pressure in terms of frequency, intensity and timing properties, and translates these fluctuations into an electrical signal that our brain can understand.

The cochlea, which looks like a snail shell, is filled with a watery liquid that moves in response to the vibrations coming from the middle ear. Thousands of hair cells sense the motion and convert that motion to electrical signals; the cochlea nerves transmit nerve impulses along the auditory nerve to the brain, which then interprets the sound waves.

Together with the cochlea (the auditory system), the vestibular system forms part of the inner ear and is mainly responsible for balance (coordination) and spatial orientation (left/right; front/back; location and directions). The vestibular system mainly sends signals to neural structures that control eye movements and balance.

You may notice this if you spin round on the spot several times and, when you stop, try to stay still and focus your eyes on a fixed point, and sense your eyes moving, trying to refocus. You may feel dizzy and even lose your balance.

Listening differs from hearing in that it takes conscious practice and effort to develop fully; it is something we consciously choose to do. Listening requires attention, interest and a desire to listen. Listening requires concentration, so that the brain processes meaning from words or sounds.

Routine hearing tests are not sufficient to diagnose an auditory processing difficulty. A child needs to be referred to an audiologist or paediatric hearing assessment for an audiogram or tympanogram test to establish any hearing sensitivity, as well as an auditory processing skills assessment to screen for and diagnose auditory processing difficulties.

You can find more information on the website for Great Ormond Street Hospital, audiology department;[20] and the Patient Information Fact Sheet from University Hospital Southampton.[21]

Retained Primitive Reflexes

This is an area of great interest to me, especially since I see many children with learning difficulties who have retained primitive reflexes and have benefited from receiving occupational therapy in the form of gentle exercises.

The UK, Sweden and Australia are leading the way in the neuro-development research into primitive reflexes and much research can be found in the *British Journal of Occupational Therapy*, the *International Journal of Special Education*, and in the world of optometry, to support theories of retained primitive reflexes interfering with academic, social, emotional, behavioural or co-ordination problems.

Retained primitive reflexes are believed to affect a child's ability to function well at school and in daily life. There is a condition known as Retained Reflex Syndrome (RRS) that many neuro specialists believe is responsible for ADHD, dyspraxia, dyslexia, autism and other learning or development problems.

There are over 70 known primary or primitive reflexes. They are automatic, involuntary movements needed for survival and development in the womb and in the early months of a baby's life. As a baby's brain develops, more mature patterns of response (called postural reflexes) develop in place of primitive reflexes. If primitive reflexes are retained past their time (i.e. not going away, or not being integrated into postural reflexes – beyond 6–12 months is considered abnormal), they can cause problems that can be linked to difficulty learning at school, such as poor eye functioning, auditory processing, poor gross or fine motor skills, sensory or emotional immaturity, attention, hyperactivity, social and behavioural issues.

Research suggests that trauma of some kind, anywhere between conception and the early months of a baby's life, may be the cause of retained primitive reflexes (such as a physical, hormonal, or chemical trauma in the womb, a traumatic prolonged birth, Caesarean section or forceps delivery). It is also suggested that stress or a traumatic event can cause integrated reflexes to 'unintegrate' at any time during a child's or adult's life.

At a primitive reflexes course called Rhythmic Movement Training,[22] I learned about how to identify whether a child or adult has unintegrated primitive reflexes, through observing body postures, symmetry and coordination. The course participants were all adults who learned how to identify my lack of body symmetry and coordination issues and were able to 'see' subtle physical issues I already knew I had with hip, neck, leg and arm discomfort on the left side of my body. I had not told anyone of these physical problems or that I had dyslexia.

The exercises I was prescribed to rectify my lack of symmetry were gentle, rhythmic and very relaxing. They were passive exercises (done by the therapist), which were effortless and very enjoyable. The active exercises needed me to focus on certain parts of my body and gently work the muscle in that area. Each exercise lasted no more than a few minutes, and I felt a general sense of well-being and relaxation afterwards. By the end of our two-day course, my body posture was already beginning to realign. Normally, when one is prescribed a programme of exercises, one does only a couple of gentle movements every day for only a few minutes, probably for about six weeks for each set of exercises. Then one is reassessed and it is likely that a new set of exercises is recommended, until the reflexes are fully integrated and the system is balanced.

It's important to note that these exercises are not a 'quick fix' and a reflex programme generally takes from six to eighteen months, depending on an individual's needs. The key is doing the movements daily for just a few minutes over several weeks or months, so as not to over stimulate the system.

The most commonly retained reflexes associated with classroom learning and learning difficulties are the Moro reflex, asymmetrical tonic neck reflex (ATNR), Spinal Galant reflex, symmetrical tonic neck reflex (STNR), tonic labyrinthine reflex (TLR) and palmar reflex.

I have also reviewed the plantar reflex, root and sucking reflex and Landau Reflex, as these are common reflexes that also affect children's and adults' physical, emotional and psychological well-being.

- The **Moro reflex** (startle reflex) acts as a baby's primitive fight or flight reaction to being startled by a sudden noise, touch or bright light. It should be inhibited by around 4 months after birth and replaced by an adult startle reflex. If it persists in children, it can be associated with not being able to control emotions, hypersensitivity to touch, light, textures, sudden changes in their surroundings, exaggerated startle reflex, being constantly in a state of alert, difficulty ignoring background noise, easily distracted, anxious, aggressive or highly excitable and can be linked to allergies.

- The **asymmetrical tonic neck reflex** (ATNR) (the 'fencing' reflex) is one of the first hand–eye co-ordination movements. It is activated as a result of turning the head to one side and the arm and leg on the same side will extend, while the opposite limbs bend. The reflex should be inhibited by 6 months of age. If the ATNR remains active for longer, the child can have difficulty crossing the midline of his body. Integration of the ATNR is crucial to good visual development. The crawling stage is extremely important in the integration of the ATNR at the right time, and children who stand and walk without crawling often experience a retained ATNR. It can lead to cross-laterality development problems, poor handwriting, difficulty completing writing tasks, difficulty walking, inattention, smooth eye movement problems, and poor balance.

- The **Spinal Galant reflex** is present at birth and should be inhibited between 3–9 months after birth. It is important for helping a baby move down the birth canal and to the development of the vestibular system, sense of balance and movement, spatial orientation, auditory processing and hearing. If it persists, it can cause restlessness (inability to sit still and remain silent), fidgeting, hyperactivity, poor concentration, poor posture and lower-back problems later in life and continued bedwetting after 5 years of age.

- The **symmetrical tonic neck reflex** (STNR) emerges after the ATNR at around 6–9 months after birth and is present in normal development until around 9–12 months after birth. The STNR helps a baby lift and control his head and is a whole-body response to movement of the neck that prepares babies for crawling. If the STNR remains present, up and down head movements remain linked to arm and leg movements, and this can affect, for example, hand to eye coordination, sitting still, walking awkwardly (ape-like walking), muscle tension, poor posture, attention span, and writing skills (such as writing on the line and in straight columns).

- The **tonic labyrinthine reflex** (TLR) is a forwards and backwards reflex and is a gradual process involving the maturation of other systems. The TLR forwards is present in the womb and ceases by around 4 months of age; the TLR backwards starts at birth and gradually completes any time between 6 weeks and 3½ years. If the TRL persists beyond this time, it can lead to poor body awareness, posture, balance and muscle tone, visual perceptual difficulties, spatial problems, motion sickness, poor sequencing skills, poor sense of direction (up/down, left/right), and difficulty judging space, distance, depth, speed or time.

- The **palmar grasp** reflex is a normal hand reflex that appears at birth and persists until 5 or 6 months of age. When an object is placed in your baby's hand or you stroke his palm, his fingers will close and he will grasp it. A retained palmar reflex can affect fine motor coordination, thumb and finger movement, cause pencil grip problems, difficulty in written expression, clumsiness and speech problems.

Other reflexes that affect children's development:

- The **plantar grasp** reflex is a normal foot reflex in babies that should be fully present at birth. It is activated by stroking the side of the sole of the foot with a sharp object, which makes the big toe (and sometimes other toes) flex. It should inhibit by 7 to 9 months of age. If the reflex is retained, known as Babinski sign, it can present difficulties with balance and coordination and learning to walk, running awkwardly, often twisting the ankle, and chronic lower back pain in adults.

- The **rooting** reflex and **suck** reflex are present at birth and should disappear by 3 to 4 months. When you stroke a baby's cheek or side of the mouth, the baby turns towards you and opens his mouth and sucks. If this reflex is retained, it may affect muscle development of the mouth and tongue, which may cause problems with swallowing, feeding, speech and manual dexterity. Some symptoms include eating noisily, messy eating, fussy eating habits due to disliking certain textures, chewing pencils and other objects, thumb sucking, poor articulation, oversensitivity to touch on the face and poor manual dexterity connected with the palmar reflex.

- The **Landau reflex** is a 'between' reflex that takes over from the TLR forwards primitive reflex and shows signs when babies reach around 4 months of age, then inhibits around 3 years and does not remain with us for life, as do postural reflexes. When a baby is held in the air and supported under its tummy, its limbs extend. If the Landau reflex is not fully integrated, the Spinal Galant may not integrate, and consequently there may be problems with development of balance due to weak muscle tone and the upper and lower parts of the body not being 'in sync'. This may manifest itself in poor posture, awkward movements in the lower body, difficulty hopping or jumping, and poor vertical eye tracking.

If you think your child has retained primitive reflexes, I suggest visiting an occupational therapist with a background in children's education who can perform a neurological assessment of these primitive reflexes. In my experience, it helps to understand what may be preventing your child from learning effectively. I highly recommend that parents are included in a reflex programme and do the exercises alongside their child, as the relaxation benefits alone are fantastic! You could make it 5 minutes of daily family fun time, so that your child doesn't feel singled out.

From a learning and self-esteem perspective, it is important to identify what is causing your child to experience difficulty in learning, such as any possible vision, hearing or physical problems and to find out which teaching methods will best help your child learn. This way, your child will have a good understanding of how he learns best, and teachers will be able to tailor teaching methods to your child's needs and preferred style of learning and provide coping strategies. I explain different styles of learning, and auditory, visual and kinaesthetic strategies to help your child learn more easily in the chapter **Learning Preferences and Multiple Intelligences**.

Chapter 6
Related learning difficulties and other conditions

That's the real problem with kids who struggle
with learning... Some kids feel like they're
stupid. I want them to know that they're not.
They just learn differently. Once they
understand that and have the tools to learn
in their individual way, then they can feel
good about themselves.

Charles Schwab, businessman[23]

I don't like identifying myself or others by 'learning disabilities'
or so-called 'disorders'. We are all unique individuals with
amazing qualities, who should not be placed into labelled
groups. Labels are not our identity. However, for educational
reasons and to get the right help for children, identifying
learning difficulties can help specialists focus on specific
strategies to help our children.

Because today's society refers to learning challenges by type,
you may wish to understand what these refer to. Therefore, in this
chapter, I look at dyspraxia, dysgraphia, dyscalculia, dysphasia
and dysnomia, five other prevalent 'dys' conditions that often
have overlapping dyslexic characteristics or indicators, known as
co-morbidity. Each of these has its own section and table
outlining the main characteristics or symptoms, to ease
identification. I also touch on other 'learning conditions', to give
you some insight and understanding, as there may be some
overlapping characteristics with dyslexia:

- Speech and Language issues
- Auditory Processing Disorder

- Visual Processing Disorder
- Sensory Processing Disorder
- Attention Deficit Hyperactivity Disorder
- Autistic Spectrum Disorder

Specific learning difficulties and dyslexia are generally due to problems with one or more of the following:

- working memory
- processing speed
- receptive and/or expressive language skills
- auditory processing
- visual processing
- organisational skills
- co-ordination skills
- maintaining concentration and attention

In my family, there are several overlapping characteristics. I have dyslexia, with difficulties in auditory processing and speech and language issues and my children have overlapping characteristics of dyslexia, speech and language and dyspraxia.

Every child is different and will display a unique set of characteristics that can be identified and better understood by having an assessment. Indeed, the degree of the difficulties will also vary and can be mild, moderate or severe in nature.

If you believe your child is displaying any of the characteristics detailed in the following sections, do not despair! These learning difficulties can be managed well with the right specialist help and early intervention.

Dyspraxia: difficulty with coordination

Dyspraxia comes under the umbrella term Developmental Coordination Disorder, or DCD. Dyspraxia characteristics are manifested in coordination skills, physical awkwardness or clumsiness. Dyspraxia may affect the gross motor muscles responsible for balance and rhythm, and posture and movement, such catching a ball, swimming, co-ordinated movement; and the fine motor muscles responsible for manual dexterity such as handwriting, dressing and hand–eye coordination tasks. Take a look at the table Brief Overview of Dyspraxia of how to recognise a child with dyspraxia. You will also find more detailed information from the **Dyspraxia Foundation**.

Brief Overview of Dyspraxia [24]

<u>The pre-school child</u>

- Is late in reaching milestones e.g. rolling over, sitting, standing, walking, and speaking
- May not be able to run, hop, jump, or catch or kick a ball although his peers can do so
- Has difficulty in keeping friends; or judging how to behave in company
- Has little understanding of concepts such as 'in', 'on', 'in front of' etc.
- Has difficulty in walking up and down stairs
- Poor at dressing
- Slow and hesitant in most actions
- Appears not to be able to learn anything instinctively but must be taught skills
- Falls over frequently
- Poor pencil grip
- Cannot do jigsaws or shape-sorting games
- Artwork is very immature
- Often anxious and easily distracted

<u>The school-age child</u>

- Probably has all the difficulties experienced by the pre-school child with dyspraxia, with little or no improvement
- Avoids PE and games

- Does badly in class but significantly better on a one-to-one basis
- Reacts to all stimuli without discrimination and attention span is poor
- May have trouble with maths and writing structured stories
- Experiences great difficulty in copying from the board
- Writes laboriously and immaturely
- Unable to remember and/or follow instructions
- Is generally poorly organised

Dyspraxia can run in families, affecting about 10% of the population, and seems to be more prevalent in males than in females. It may be seen in a large number of children with Asperger Syndrome, and may overlap with dysgraphia, dyslexia, dyscalculia, attention deficit hyperactivity disorder (ADD/ADHD) or autism.

As with dyslexia, dyspraxia may be diagnosed as mild, moderate or severe. A person with severe dyspraxia may also have poor organisational skills, trouble with perception, and speech and language issues. He may also suffer from poor short-term memory or speed of processing. Other characteristics include sensitivity to light or sound, poor visual perception and difficulty focusing from one thing to another, such as looking up from a book to watch the television. In conversation, people with dyspraxia may interrupt others or be difficult to understand. Children with severe dyspraxia can sometimes be messy, unfocused, erratic and easily distracted.

Having dyspraxia can lead to educational underachievement if it is not diagnosed and addressed. I first recommend an educational assessment, which would then recommend a clinical assessment by an occupational therapist if necessary.

Dysgraphia: difficulty with handwriting

Handwriting problems are often present in children because of immaturity in the neurological pathways involved in the coordination of eye, hand, arm and head movements. This immaturity is confirmed by the presence of an asymmetrical tonic neck reflex (ATNR) in school-aged children. The ATNR is a primitive reflex, normally present in a full-term newborn, which is inhibited as the brain develops in the first six months of post-natal life.

A retained ATNR in an older child can result in difficulties in learning how to write. This is because, when a child's head turns to follow the direction of the writing hand, the arm and hand want to extend and the fingers want to open, making it difficult to hold on to the pencil. As a result, some children learn to compensate by using an immature pencil grip, with the result that holding and working a pencil for any length of time requires great effort. This can lead to an unnatural pencil grip that can cause tension in the body. In effect, the child concentrates so hard on writing that he is distracted from the writing content.

Retention of the ATNR can result in writing problems in the absence of reading difficulties or other specific learning difficulties, and is considered a specific form of dysgraphia. Take a look at the section on **Retained Primitive Reflexes**.

Dysgraphia is manifested by letters that may vary in size and shape, inconsistent letter formation, mixing up cursive and non-cursive writing and is generally hard to read. It is caused by poor muscle sequencing or muscle memory used in fine motor skills. Dysgraphia is often present alongside other learning difficulties such as dyspraxia.

In my experience, handwriting is a complex skill for many children to acquire, and poor handwriting will often result in poor spelling and can lead to academic underachievement. I see many seven-year-olds with handwriting difficulties due to incorrect pencil grip and weaknesses in fine motor control that could have been prevented with timely intervention. Correct pencil grip, i.e. the tripod grip, may not seem terribly important when they are very young and learning to write, but for some children it can be fundamental to their success in education.

Incorrect pencil grip, poor letter formation and non-cursive handwriting will have an effect on the speed of writing, which becomes particularly important when they are older, e.g. when taking notes in class or sitting exams. Children who do not use the tripod grip when drawing or writing may suffer from tension in their fingers, hand, wrist, arm, shoulders and neck, which may cause writing fatigue, headaches and lead to stress. It is extremely difficult for children to change their pencil grip after the age of 6 or 7, because it entails changing the motor memory. It can be achieved with much perseverance but is often a difficult task and best done with a specialist.

You may have come across varying terms that professionals use to describe dysgraphia, which can be somewhat confusing. Dr Linda Silverman, an expert in learning difficulties and handwriting, refers to different professions using different terminology when referring to handwriting difficulties. Special educators refer to it as dysgraphia, occupational therapists call it sensory-motor integration dysfunction, optometrists say it is visual-motor impairment, and psychologists refer to it as developmental coordination disorder (DCD).[25]

In her research paper Poor Handwriting: A Major Cause of Underachievement, Dr Silverman has composed a diagnostic checklist of writing disabilities.[26] Every child is unique and, therefore, may exhibit a combination of the symptoms in the table. If your child exhibits more than half of these symptoms, I recommend having a comprehensive assessment.

Characteristics of Dysgraphia
Diagnostic checklist of writing disabilities[27]
• Is his writing posture awkward? (like a scrunched up pretzel)
• Does he hold his pencil strangely?
• Can you see the tension run through his hand, arm, furrowed brow?
• Does it take him much longer to write than anyone else his age?
• Does he fatigue easily and want to quit? (Are you hearing a lot of groans?)
• Does he space his letters on the paper in an unusual way (too close, too far apart, no spaces between words)?

- Does he form his letters oddly (e.g., starting letters at the top that others would start at the bottom and vice versa)?
- Does he mix upper and lower case letters?
- Does he mix cursive and manuscript?
- Are his cursive letters disconnected?
- Does he prefer manuscript to cursive?
- Does his lettering lack fluidity (looks sort of like chicken-scratching)?
- Does he still reverse letters after age 7?
- Is his handwriting illegible?
- Is his spelling terrible?
- Does he avoid writing words he can't spell?
- Does he leave off the endings of words?
- Does he confuse singulars and plurals?
- Does he mix up small words, like "the" and "they"?
- Does he leave out soft sounds, like the "d" in gardener?
- Is his grasp of phonics weak? (Is it difficult to decipher what he was trying to spell?)

Dyscalculia: difficulty with numbers and maths

Dyscalculia is a difference in brain function that makes it difficult to grasp the concepts of time and direction, as well as difficulty with numbers and maths. It is important to emphasise that a general low ability in maths does not constitute dyscalculia.

As with dyspraxia and dyslexia, there are varying degrees from mild to severe and not all people with dyscalculia will manifest all the characteristics to the same degree. Characteristics of dyscalculia can show up sporadically and be inconsistent. A child may appear to have no difficulty one day and on another day be unable to do simple arithmetic.

As dyscalculia and dyslexia have similar and overlapping characteristics, it is sometimes difficult to distinguish the source of the difficulty. Not all dyslexic learners have trouble with maths and not all dyscalculic learners have trouble with reading and writing. It is estimated that about 50–60% of children with dyslexia do have difficulties with maths. The fact reading and writing are difficult for dyslexic learners makes maths harder, since they must read the maths problems, decode the words, and sequence the maths operations in the correct order. Poor short-term memory or speed of processing may affect children with either condition.

As yet, there is no definitive test to diagnose dyscalculia. However, the *Symptoms of Dyscalculia* by Dr Anna Wilson[28] in the table will help you identify if your child has dyscalculic tendencies. The **Numeracy Skills** chapter provides more in-depth information about acquiring number skills.

Symptoms of Dyscalculia

1. Delay in counting. Five– to seven-year-old dyscalculic children show less understanding of basic counting principles than their peers (e.g. that it doesn't matter which order objects are counted in).

2. Delay in using counting strategies for addition. Dyscalculic children tend to keep using inefficient strategies for calculating addition facts much longer than their peers.

3. Difficulties in memorising arithmetic facts. Dyscalculic children have great difficulty in memorising simple addition, subtraction and multiplication facts (e.g. 5 + 4 = 9), and this difficulty persists up to at least the age of thirteen.

These symptoms may be caused by two more fundamental difficulties, although more research is needed to be sure:

Lack of 'number sense'. Dyscalculic children may have a fundamental difficulty in understanding quantity. They are slower at even very simple quantity tasks such as comparing two numbers (which is bigger, 7 or 9?), and saying how many there are for groups of 1–3 objects. The brain areas which appear to be affected in dyscalculia are areas which are specialised to represent quantity.

---

4. Less automatic processing of written numbers. In most of us, reading the symbol '7' immediately causes our sense of quantity to be accessed. In dyscalculic individuals this access appears to be slower and more effortful. Thus dyscalculic children may have difficulty in linking written or spoken numbers to the idea of quantity.

Other symptoms

If you have read other websites on dyscalculia you may have seen quite a few other symptoms listed. Many of these are not yet proved to be symptoms (although this does not mean they might not be later on). This is because they have been reported by teachers or special education workers, but haven't yet been studied in detail by researchers. The following are likely to be symptoms of dyscalculia:

1. Difficulty imagining a mental number line
2. Particular difficulty with subtraction
3. Difficulty using finger counting (slow, inaccurate, unable to immediately recognise finger configurations)
4. Difficulty decomposing numbers (e.g. recognising that 10 is made up of 4 and 6)
5. Difficulty understanding place value
6. Trouble learning and understanding reasoning methods and multi-step calculation procedures
7. Anxiety about or negative attitude towards maths (caused by the dyscalculia!)
8. All these symptoms (bar the last) are related to quantity.

Dysphasia: difficulty with language

Dysphasia is a delay in speech and language and a difficulty in comprehension or verbal expression. It may affect understanding, speaking, reading or writing. Dysphasia can be receptive or expressive. Receptive dysphasia is difficulty understanding word meaning and spoken language, whereas expressive dysphasia is difficulty in putting words together to make meaning and to express thoughts and feelings.

Children with dysphasia need encouragement and support with their communication. Give your child plenty of time to speak, make sure there is no background noise or distraction, and show patience and understanding. A speech and language therapist can diagnose dysphasia and put together a programme to help your child. You can also read more in the Speech and Language section following. Some *Characteristics of Dysphasia* are listed in the summary table.

Characteristics of Dysphasia
• May understand speech well (receptive), better than speaking (expressive)
• Speech may not be completely understandable
• Speech may not be fluent or may be hesitant
• Sometimes spontaneous speech is better than in a conversation, because he is put on the spot during a dialogue
• Seems to miss the point or confused by what is being said
• Reading comprehension difficulties
• Difficulty with grammatical structure
• May find connecting ideas difficult, such as telling stories
• Difficulty writing or doing numerical calculations

Dysnomia: difficulty finding words or recalling names

Most people have a balance between receptive language (the ability to understand, retain and integrate knowledge) and expressive language (to put it into words). Children with dysnomia have a far higher level of receptive language than expressive language. Dysnomia is a noticeable difficulty in remembering names or recalling a word needed for spoken or written language. It is like a severe form of the 'tip-of-the-tongue' feeling, where the brain cannot recall the desired word or name. Dyslexia can overlap with dysnomia because of word retrieval similarities.

Doctors diagnose dysnomia when neuropsychological tests show a significantly greater than normal difficulty recalling words or names. This is a medical condition when severe enough to interfere with daily life. Dysnomia is a lesser level of impairment than anomia (being completely unable to name familiar objects). When your child is trying to find words: give him time to try and recall names and help him if he gets stuck. A speech and language therapist can assess your child and put together a language programme and recall exercises to reinforce vocabulary. *Characteristics of Dysnomia* are listed below.

Characteristics of Dysnomia

- Trouble remembering names, places, objects, words or numbers
- Speaking hesitantly because of difficulty naming words
- Having good knowledge of an object, but being unable to name it
- Replacing a word with a synonym because they cannot remember the word they want to use
- Reading ability may be impaired
- Writing ability may be impaired
- Levels of comprehension are not affected

Other learning difficulties and learning disorders

Speech and language difficulties

Speech and language difficulties fall into two categories: receptive and expressive. Receptive language refers to meaning, understanding and 'decoding' language. Expressive language refers to production, spoken output and coding (a process of formulating ideas into words and sentences). Any child who has difficulty understanding language will have difficulty expressing himself.

Earlier, I talked about phonemic awareness and the difficulty that dyslexic learners often have with recognising sounds. This difficulty may extend to the spoken as well as the written language. Sometimes this results in slurred or indistinct speech or word retrieval problems, and this can be especially true when there is also evidence of verbal dyspraxia.

When identifying a speech and language problem, I would recommend first a specialist teacher or educational psychologist assessment to obtain an overall understanding of your child. As part of your child's assessment, the recommendations may include a speech and language assessment.

Difficulties with speech and language are not necessarily the result of dyslexia but could be the result of many different conditions. If speech is a problem, your child's educational/school psychologist or speech therapist may also want to work with an audiologist, who can check for hearing loss. It is important to identify the exact reason for the speech difficulty, to help your child overcome it.

Speech therapy may take the form of training to help your child listen to and distinguish between certain sounds. The speech therapist may introduce exercises to assist with articulation, especially any sounds your child is having particular difficulty with ('th', 'v' and 'f' are common confusions).

The ability to articulate well requires the physical parts of the body to work properly, but it is also the result of being able to observe and distinguish sounds in other people's speech. Syntax or grammar is acquired through education and through reading. Together, articulation and good grammar are key to mastering language comprehension, speaking the language effectively and developing sound communication skills.

Some children with dyslexia may have trouble ordering words in a sentence as they speak or in finding the right words to use. They may mispronounce words or forget their meaning until they become very familiar with them. They may also have trouble understanding or remembering what others are saying. In severe cases, children may practise selective mutism, which means they may just decide to stop talking in some situations to avoid the pain or embarrassment that comes from not being able to master the language.

Some children may have more obvious signs of speech and language problems such as a stutter or stammer. It used to be thought that not focusing on a child stuttering and drawing attention to the problem would cause it, eventually, to go away. According to Caroline Bowen PhD:[29]

> Pretending to ignore a stutter... or pretending that stuttering is a normal phase in speech and language development is completely the wrong thing to do. It may leave the child confused and wondering why his struggle to speak fluently is an unmentionable subject.

I know of several adults whose parents believed their child would 'grow out' of a stutter and did not seek help, and I'm afraid their stutter did not go away. Early intervention is best, so seek advice and reassurance from a speech and language therapist as early as possible. For further information, see **www.rcslt.org** and in the **Appendix** for websites across the world.

Auditory processing disorder (APD)

In order to distinguish words or sounds, our brain has to interpret the sounds that are heard through the ear. Children with Auditory Processing Disorder (APD) are not deaf or of partial hearing, but their central nervous system (CNS) is unable to interpret sounds efficiently. APD is also referred to as CAPD, Central Auditory Processing Disorder.

In the classroom, children may have difficulty expressing themselves clearly; difficulty understanding when someone is speaking, especially if they talk too fast or too quietly; trouble understanding what is being read or remembering instructions, or concentrating. For example, it is possible your child may read fluently but be unable to process and make sense of the information he is reading. Lack of comprehension may be manifested in a difficulty recapping a story line or answering questions about a text.

Not all learning, language and communication deficits are due to APD. It is an auditory disorder that is not the result of higher-order global deficits, such as autism, mental retardation, attention deficits or similar impairments. APD cannot be diagnosed from a checklist of symptoms and is a difficult disorder to detect and diagnose. Diagnosis should be made by a multi-disciplinary team, and may initially be picked up by a specialist teacher or educational psychologist, who will recommend further investigation by an audiologist. The audiologist will use a selection of tests that use both simple auditory stimuli such as tones, noise bursts and clicks, and other complex stimuli such as speech. For further information see **Auditory processing problems** (previous chapter) or go to **www.apduk.org.uk** or **www.capdsupport.org**.

Visual processing disorder

A visual processing difficulty, or visual perception processing disorder, affects how the brain perceives visual information and processes what the eye can see. It can affect gross and fine motor skills due to problems with eye to hand coordination.

In the classroom, children may have difficulty with literacy or maths. They may reverse letters or numbers; skip words or lines when reading; find it difficult to read at speed and accurately; find copying from the board difficult; have problems writing neatly; find judging distance difficult; and have difficulty noticing the similarities and differences between letters, colours, patterns, shapes and symbols.

Initially, an educational psychologist or specialist teacher may pick up on difficulties during an educational assessment and recommend that your child be assessed by an optometrist who will perform a behavioural vision assessment. For more information see **Visual processing problems** (previous chapter).

Sensory processing disorder (SPD)

Sensory processing disorder (SPD) or sensory integration disorder/dysfunction (SID) is a neurological disorder that affects how effectively and efficiently a person is able to process sensory information from one or more of the following senses: visual (looking), auditory (hearing), olfactory (smell), gustatory (taste), tactile (touch), vestibular (movement), proprioceptive (body position and sense of one's limbs in space).

Sensory signals are not organised into appropriate responses and a child may have significant difficulty processing information, which may affect daily functioning such as behaviour, family and social relationships, regulation of emotions, learning and self-esteem. SPD varies between people in their characteristics and intensity. Some people are so mildly afflicted that the disorder is hardly noticeable; while others are so impaired they have trouble with daily functioning.

Children can be born hypersensitive or hyposensitive to varying degrees and may have trouble in one sense, a few, or all the senses. Hypersensitivity includes feeling pain from clothing rubbing against skin, an inability to tolerate normal lighting in a room, a dislike of being touched (especially light touch) and discomfort when looking directly into the eyes of another person. Hyposensitivity is characterised by an unusually high tolerance for environmental stimuli. A child with hyposensitivity might appear restless and seek sensory stimulation.

It is important to be assessed by an occupational therapist (OT), who will produce a sensory diet programme with a Sensory Integration (SI) approach. Sometimes, listening therapy or other complementary therapies may be combined with OT-SI. There are many signs and symptoms of SPD according to the sense affected, and you will find excellent information on the SPD website: **www.sensory-processing-disorder.com**.

Attention deficit disorder with or without hyperactivity (ADHD/ADD)

ADD is commonly used to refer to attention deficit disorder without hyperactivity. It is an old term: the official name is now attention deficit hyperactivity disorder, inattentive type. ADHD is used to describe attention deficit disorder with hyperactivity. Both are considered to be a type of the same condition, but there are some major differences.

Children with ADD have trouble focusing and concentrating, but are not hyperactive. Typically, they have very weak short-term/working memories. In the classroom, they may not talk or move around too much or get into trouble for poor behaviour. But, because they find it very difficult to focus, they may miss out on what is being taught. Other times, children appear to be paying attention but can be thinking about many things besides their school work.

Children with ADHD are very busy, always on the go. They are hyperactive, move around a lot, need to fidget or tap, and like getting up and down. They are impulsive, often doing things without thinking of the consequences, and may experience mood swings. They are usually inattentive and find staying focused very challenging, especially on tasks that are not immediately rewarding.

In the classroom, they are often in trouble for moving around/talking too much, tapping their pencil on their desk or getting up without permission to sharpen their pencil and so forth. This behaviour is consistent over long periods. A child who is restless sometimes or fidgety does not necessarily have ADHD. However, a child who is never able to concentrate on sitting still is a possible candidate. Some children are more inattentive than hyperactive and others are more hyperactive. Some are a combination of both.

Having ADD or ADHD prevents children from concentrating normally, and affects their social and educational development. It is thought to be an inherited condition and affects more boys than girls, though it can affect both.

Some theories suggest that ADHD is the result of differences in genes that regulate important chemicals in the brain: *dopamine* (plays an important role in behaviour, learning, mood, dependency, positive reinforcement), *serotonin* (responsible for mood, digestion, appetite, sleep, pain, regulating body temperature), *norepinephrine* (important for attentiveness, alertness, learning, emotions, sleeping, dreaming) and *melatonin* (a sleep hormone made by *serotonin*, normally secreted at night, which regulates energy balance, body weight and sex hormone production). It is believed that low levels of *serotonin* in the brain contribute to ADD and high levels contribute to ADHD.

Children who are diagnosed with ADHD may have other learning difficulties such as dyslexia or dyspraxia. If left unmanaged, the condition can give rise to serious behavioural problems, such as oppositional defiant disorder, and will prevent your child from learning effectively. When diagnosed early, there are effective alternative therapies, natural diets and natural medications that can help children overcome the disorder. Children prefer a bodily-kinaesthetic style of learning that enables them to move about a bit. In my experience, many children with ADHD are very talented, wonderfully creative, have fun, amusing personalities and plenty of friends. Is it surprising with all that amazing energy? For further information go to **www.addiss.co.uk** or **www.chadd.org**.

Autistic spectrum disorder (ASD)

Autism is another form of developmental disorder that can take several forms. It is called autism spectrum disorder or ASD, because it covers a spectrum of difficulties that are not always present in all cases. Asperger Syndrome is a form of autism. The three main areas that might be impacted are social interaction, social communication and social imagination.

Autism can be difficult to recognise and diagnose. Many sufferers simply appear a little different or difficult to get along with and may be ignored or bullied by their peers, while inside they are struggling to understand social interactions. A multi-disciplinary team of professionals, such as a paediatrician, psychiatrist, speech and language therapist, occupational therapist and clinical psychologist, should make a formal assessment.

Autism causes people to struggle with communication and interaction on a social level, and people with autism suffer a great deal of stress and anxiety when they have to deal with people on an individual level or in a crowd. Even everyday family interactions can be hard for them.

At school, and at home, many children with autism prefer to be alone rather than with others. They have trouble expressing emotions, emotional needs and feelings. They may have few friends.

Children benefit from having structure and routine in their life, which helps them feel secure. They need to know that things are going to be predictable, so that they can deal with them. Change can be very intimidating since they lack organisational and imagination skills.

People with autism find it hard to understand body language. When you frown or make a face to indicate dislike, disapproval, pleasure and so on, children with autism are unlikely to understand. They will take what you say literally, often missing the point of a double-entendre, joke or sarcastic comment.

Some children with severe autism may have trouble speaking. Some choose not to speak at all, while others seem not to have difficulty speaking and yet be awkward or clumsy in conversation, not understanding the natural rhythm of give and take that occurs when people talk.

Another manifestation of autism can be extremely sensitive skin. Some people with autism cannot bear to feel their clothing against their skin, and clothes made of rough or restricting fabrics can be irritating and cause distress. They can also be sensitive to sounds, lights and smells.

It can be alarming to find out that your child has autism. Talk to other parents and go to support groups, which are a great source of advice, comfort and understanding of what you are all going through. Share what does and doesn't work for your child and your family. For further information go to the National Autistic Society **www.autism.org.uk**.

Responding to children's behaviour

It is not only vital to discover the reason for children having difficulty learning, it is also imperative to get help for children who behave badly. It is rare that a young child or teenager behaves badly for no reason. You and teachers need to play detective until you find the cause.

**We need to be patient with our children,
and we need to be patient with ourselves**

Parents of children with severe learning difficulties, extreme behaviour or obsessive tendencies need to dig deep to find the patience and understanding these children need. Many children feel sad, stressed out and inadequate because they are not understood, which consequently affects their mood, behaviour and well-being. Alternative therapies, relaxation techniques, music, art, play and sound therapies all play a special role in relieving stress, tension and sad emotions.

In my experience, while some of children's difficulties can be tough and exhausting to manage, our children are often smart and display positive qualities and amazing talents. We must be patient with them, and with ourselves. Your child's tireless daydreaming, wonderful imagination or high energy makes him innovative and exciting. A great way to manage the behaviour is by helping him discover, unleash and channel his talents and energy.

Education is not filling a bucket,
but lighting a fire.[30]

Chapter 7
Our memory and memory strategies

We remember what we understand; we understand only what we pay attention to; we pay attention to what we want.

Edmund Blair Bolles, science writer[31]

Memory is the essence of learning; it exists on both conscious and unconscious levels and is fundamental to the learning process. There are three major processes involved in memory: encoding, storage and retrieval. Memory begins with perception of information, which first enters our memory through one or more of our senses (sensory stage). Information is then transferred into our short-term working memory and until we have stored it safely in our long-term memory, we haven't 'learned' it.

We all experience occasions of remembering what may seem irrelevant facts, yet struggle to remember information at school. As Tom Cruise learned to train himself to focus his attention, many of us also have to train our memories to remember certain information.

Let's see how our memory works in more detail.

How our memory works

Memory is more than a concept. It is a physical characteristic of the human brain. It has been proved in countless studies that, while many people with dyslexia have dependable and often very good long-term memories, they may typically have inefficient short-term/working memories, which makes the learning process at school more difficult for them.

Take a look at the picture of our brain. Information first enters our sensory memory through our main sensory organs of touch, sight, hearing, taste and smell, as we read, listen to and perceive new information. The sensory memory is very short term: information is held there for only a few milliseconds.

Information passes from the sensory memory to the short-term memory, also called the working memory, because it is where we process information before we decide what to discard and what to move to long-term memory.

The short-term memory is located in an area of our brain called the pre-frontal lobe, which is located right behind our forehead. Much of the information that enters our short-term memory is forgotten immediately, especially if it does not resonate with us, or strike any chords of familiarity. Later in this chapter, I talk more about the 'forgetting curve'. Below is a memory model originally conceived by Baddeley and Hitch[32], which I have simplified and adapted. It illustrates how information is processed by the brain into our sensory memory, working memory and long-term memory.

Sensory Memory, Working Memory and Long-term Memory Process

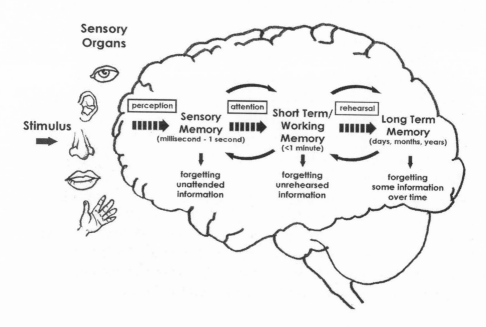

Under certain conditions, information is transferred to long-term memory. If something strikes us as unusually interesting or compelling, we are more likely to remember it (the 'von Restorff effect'). Named after Hedwig von Restorff, this is also called the 'isolation effect'. It predicts that information or experiences that 'stand out like a sore thumb' (called distinctive encoding) are more likely to be remembered than other experiences, i.e. if we make a learning experience memorable, it is more likely to make an impact on us and be remembered.

After a few seconds or minutes, information either leaves the short-term memory, dropping out into the forgotten zone, or is moved to long-term memory. Interestingly, information that is already in our long-term memory is a significant factor in how much we retain from our short-term memory, because we often need related information from long-term memory to understand or process information in our short-term memory.

Short-term memory/working memory

Information enters your short-term memory through your senses and also from using your imagination, thinking, remembering and intuition. Your short-term memory holds the information for typically 10-30 seconds, or even up to a minute (the exact amount of time varies depending on your physical characteristics, which are different for everyone). For people with dyslexia, this time is likely to be shorter, sometimes only a few seconds or less.

The short-term memory is not just for absorbing new information. It is also called working memory because it is a storage area for information that you recall from your long-term memory to help process new information.

Most of us can store several pieces of information in our short-term memory at a time but, if we try to cram too much into it, our memory becomes overwhelmed and we lose information quickly. It used to be thought that seven was the magic number of items we could store in our memories.[33] However, studies by various psychologists indicate that the number can vary between three and ten depending on the person.

Psychologists have also studied the amount of spoken information we can remember. This number ranges from about one and a half to two seconds. Again, the exact amount you remember depends on how fast the speaker is speaking and the physical characteristics of your memory. The memory that listens to the spoken word is called the 'phonological loop'.

To move information from your short-term memory to your long-term memory, you have to act quickly before you forget it. There are various ways to do this, and sometimes the act is unconscious. Other times you have to work at it.

Moving information from short-term to long-term memory

When we process new information that is in our short-term memory, we use (usually subconscious) processes to move information that strikes us as interesting, amusing and informative to our long-term memories. Information that fails to capture our attention is filtered out almost immediately. If we don't make a conscious effort to remember information, it can gradually fade over a few seconds or, for some of us, it can disappear suddenly.

The NTL Institute for Applied Behavioural Science (National Training Laboratory) in Maine has researched average student retention rates of information after 24 hours. It makes for interesting reinforcement of using a combination of visual, auditory and kinaesthetic (VAK) learning styles.

The research reports that we remember only about 5% of a lecture and 10% of what we read. However, if we discuss it within a group (engaging our verbal and auditory senses), we are likely to remember five times as much.

Likewise, if we also make notes as we listen to a lecture or read, or we physically play around with sentences and words, we engage additional senses, which helps to move the information into long-term memory. Consequently, we are likely to remember a great deal more. More than that, having a written record gives us a memory tool to refer back to. If we 'feel' what we read, we are more likely to remember it too.

If students teach others what they have learned or use the learned information straightaway, they are likely to retain 90% after 24 hours.

People with dyslexia who are successful in overcoming the shortcomings of short-term memory learn to make good use of multi-sensory learning.

Average retention rate after 24 hours

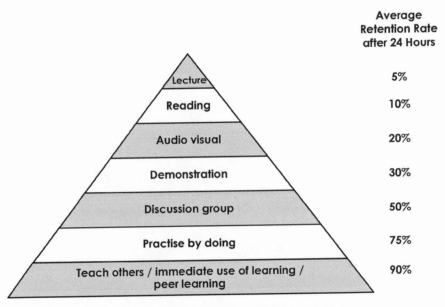

Average Retention Rate after 24 Hours

Lecture	5%
Reading	10%
Audio visual	20%
Demonstration	30%
Discussion group	50%
Practise by doing	75%
Teach others / immediate use of learning / peer learning	90%

Source: NTL Institute for Applied Behavioural Science. (National Training Laboratory), Maine

Long-term memory

The part of the brain responsible for moving information from short-term to long-term memory is called the hippocampus. We have several different kinds of long-term memory,[34] such as episodic memory, semantic memory, procedural memory, spatial memory and emotional memory. Each of these is located in different areas of the brain. The hippocampus acts as a sort of broker to decide which part of our memory to route the new information to.

Much study has been done about the physiological aspect of human memory for people with and without dyslexia; so we know a lot about which physical parts of the brain come into play when we use our memory for different things. For example, we use different parts of memory to store important information, such as our own address, remembering how to ride a bike, remembering a number for a short time to do a simple addition problem and so on. Our knowledge of the way the memory works is not just theoretical but is backed up by numerous laboratory studies that have used magnetic resonance imaging (MRI) technology to map activity in the brain.

The information in long-term memory impacts on what we can remember. If a concept is familiar, it is easier to remember new information because we associate it with information we have already learned on that subject.

Let's say you are trying to remember the colours of the rainbow. If you have already seen a rainbow and hold the image in your long-term memory, it will be easier to remember the colours. When you learn that red is one of the colours, you will remember what red looks like, and you will be able to associate the red colour with the red band in a rainbow. If you have never seen a rainbow, and you have never seen the colour red, it will be much harder to remember that red is a colour in the rainbow.

Our brains are constantly using information already known to process new information. This is why you can read a text passage to a class full of children and some will remember some things, while others will remember different things about the text.

Dyslexia and memory

Dyslexic learners have a different way of processing information. They may be holistic thinkers and process information using all their senses and may look at things from a non-linear, big-picture perspective. Dyslexic thinkers are often creative and can handle complex thoughts and ideas but may not do well with a traditional, linear approach to problem solving that is rooted in the written word. This is why pictures, colour coding, spider graphs, Mind Maps®, verbalising and visualising and other visual impact tools are very effective for people with dyslexia.

Many parents, including me, say that their child has a 'great memory', so we find it very hard to understand that their short-term memory might be weak and that they have problems remembering information at school.

When children fail to carry out simple instructions, or forget to brush their teeth before going to school or to do a homework assignment, it is easy to attribute their behaviour to other things, such as being lazy or unreliable. This confusion is compounded by the fact that children with dyslexia often exhibit above-average intelligence, very good long-term memories and are interested in many different topics; yet have difficulty with simple tasks such as remembering to bring a textbook home, copying information from the whiteboard or picking up their jacket when leaving the bus.

Your child is every bit as frustrated and confused as you are at not being able to remember day-to-day things

It is frustrating arriving at school only to find you left your lunchbox on the kitchen counter yet again, or don't know whether to turn left or right at the end of the hallway to reach your next classroom. It is embarrassing going to visit your friend and ending up at the wrong house because you switched the house number from 34 to 43. Your child is every bit as frustrated and confused as you are at not being able to remember day-to-day things.

Many don't recognise poor memory as the problem. Instead, some people may assume that children who are slow learners are of lower intelligence – this is not the case. Today, many schools implement testing for dyslexia at around age seven or eight but, at this age, some children may already have been left behind in terms of the school curriculum. A study conducted at Durham University[35] looked at over 3,000 children and found that 10% had poor working memory. An outcome of this study was the development of the Working Memory Rating Scale, or WMRS. It is used to identify children with working memory deficit from 5 to 11 years of age and is already being used in schools in many countries.

Your child with dyslexia will not grow out of having a poor working memory, but it is not a sign of low intelligence. It is a physical characteristic your child most likely inherited. While there is no 'cure' for a short-term memory problem, it is possible to help your child train his memory to perform better; and you can teach him a variety of tips, tricks and coping strategies that will help him remember information or instructions.

The benefit of having an educational assessment cannot be overestimated in the short and long term: both at school and for future career choice. Children with learning difficulties are more likely to have an educational assessment than their counterparts. Not only will an educational assessment highlight children's challenges, which can be managed through the development of learning strategies, but also what they are good at. This is highly beneficial for a child's self-esteem and self-awareness. Many children leave school unaware of what they are good at, but children who are fully aware of their strengths can make better-informed choices about their working life. This in turn provides greater job satisfaction, avoids job burnout and results in a happier and more fulfilled life.

My children know their strengths and weaknesses inside out. They understand what they find difficult, and use coping strategies to overcome their memory and other difficulties; but they also know what they are good at. This self-knowledge, which was triggered by having an educational assessment, helped them choose university courses and careers that were in harmony with their strengths and personalities.

Forgetting, oops!

One of the hardest parts of remembering is overcoming our natural tendency to forget! That might sound like stating the obvious but you may not realise that forgetting is a natural part of the brain's processing and a certain amount of forgetting is always going to happen.

Experts think we do most of our forgetting immediately after we learn something. Because the short-term memory fades very quickly, we have to work at moving it to the long-term memory in a variety of ways.

Herman Ebbinghaus studied memory in the late 1800s and came up with a graph known as the Forgetting Curve,[36] which illustrates just how quickly we lose information from our working memory. Within an hour of learning something new, we typically forget about 50% of it. Within nine hours we forget about 60% and after a month we have forgotten about 80%. We can improve these numbers by a steady focus on remembering and by using a number of different memory strategies.

After a number of days, the amount of information you forget declines more gradually and eventually levels off. Whatever information you still remember after about a month you are likely to remember a lot longer.

Automaticity

On the other side of the forgetting curve is a concept we call 'automaticity'. If we continuously repeat an action, it becomes ingrained in our brains and we are able to repeat it without consciously thinking about it.

Another way to think of this is when you have become so familiar with something that you can perform it on 'autopilot'. Have you driven home from work and been unable to remember anything about your journey, including which way you took and what the traffic was like? That is an example of automaticity in action. You are so familiar with driving your route, operating the vehicle, watching the traffic and obeying the traffic signals, that you managed to do it without a thought, as your mind was busy thinking over a problem you had at work, or something you needed to sort out at home.

Automaticity is also the principle at play when experts master difficult tasks such as an orbital analyst performing a complex calculation or a virtuoso pianist performing a difficult concerto. Scientists believe that automaticity occurs when we perform an action in a carefully controlled way, gradually building upon it, adding more complexity over time. Each time we perform the action, we are moving information from our working memory into our long-term memory.

When we learn to drive a car, for example, we don't go out on a busy road right away. First, we master the controls, turning the key in the ignition, moving the gear lever, and accelerating slowly before we build up speed. Once we pass our test, we don't automatically know the way to get to places. We get lost and we use maps and signs, and eventually we know exactly where the local roads go and how to get to the shops, to work, and so on.

When we have completely mastered something, the demand on our conscious mind is less and we can do things automatically. Another word for it is 'over-learning'.

People with dyslexia might need to work harder at remembering small things but, once they achieve over-learning, it is locked in their long-term memory and becomes easier. They accomplish over-learning by constant repetition, which is why I can't emphasise enough the importance of constant practice and repetition, even at small things such as spelling a difficult word or repeating a times table until it is locked in the memory.

Over-learning improves automatic recall

No matter which strategy we choose to remember something, effective learning takes place when we repeat and practise it over and over until it is truly embedded into our long-term memories and past the point in the forgetting curve where we are still vulnerable to forgetting it. When we have learned something thoroughly, recalling it becomes automatic. This is the case with learning the sounds of the alphabet, times tables, telephone numbers or any other common fact we use in our daily lives and need to recall repeatedly during the course of a day.

Children with dyslexia have to work harder than most to accomplish automatic recall of information (automaticity)

It used to be thought that memory is like a muscle, and must be exercised regularly like other parts of the body.[37] Those with poor memory were thought of as academically lazy. This belief was gradually replaced with the theory that memory is more or less a genetic condition that can be inherited. You are blessed biologically with either a good memory or a bad one and, if you were allotted a bad memory, there was nothing much you could do about it.

Today, a more popular belief is somewhere in the middle. Some people have better athletic ability than others, but those who are naturally the fastest runners can improve their competitive edge by intensive training. Some are naturally gifted musicians and become extraordinary experts, whereas others can learn to play the piano or another instrument well enough to become performers if they apply themselves to learning their scales and arpeggios. It is now widely accepted that much the same thing is true of memory. Some are naturally gifted with wonderful memories and others are not, but those with poor memories can do much to improve memory retention by regular training and dedication to applying the right techniques for learning.

I know from first-hand experience that there are ways you can help your child make substantial progress. You need to help your child figure out what strategies work best for him, as what works for some people does not work for others. Try a few things and see what works best. Sooner or later your child will figure out personalised learning strategies and ways of remembering and learning, but at the start will need much help and patience on your part.

So is it possible to improve our memory? According to many scientists, yes it is, and according to others, it isn't! Many believe our memory can be honed and sharpened with the right lifestyle (holistic) choices and a basic knowledge of memory-enhancing strategies.

Look at the following memory strategies section with your child and talk about the approaches that work best for your child's personality and circumstances.

Strategies and techniques for successful memorisation

Best time to remember

Some studies suggest the best time of day for remembering is in the afternoon.[38] Others suggest last thing at night or during your sleep! However, I am a morning person and this is when I am at my most alert and focused, so I revise in the morning, review the information in the afternoon and again the following morning. The aim is for repetition, little and often. So, when remembering information is really important, read it over, recite it out loud a few times, write it down, draw visual Mind Maps® or other methods detailed below, then review it again before you go to bed, and again first thing in the morning. You will notice quite a difference in being able to recall this information if you practise the repetition and review technique.

Once we understand the physical nature of memory and how long-term memory is important for short-term memory, it is easy to see the most important part of learning successfully is to make sure that information gets into your long-term memory. The easiest way to make this happen can be summed in three words:

Repetition, repetition, repetition

In the following pages, I give several techniques and strategies for moving information from short-term to long-term memory. These are effective strategies for learning that work even for people with very poor short-term memories. There are two basic strategies for remembering, described below.

Rote learning

Rote learning is learning something by repeating it over and over. You usually apply rote learning in a sequential fashion (in order), so when you learn the alphabet, you learn the beginning letters first and the ending letters last, building upon the sequence a letter at a time until you remember the whole thing. Rote learning works well for remembering small items such as names, addresses and phone numbers, but it is not an effective way to store large amounts of information in your brain. You practise rote learning when you say the times tables over many times in order to remember them (as we did at school).

Elaborative rehearsal

This is a complicated way of expressing the fact that you think about what you are learning. One way to do that is to link new material to information you already know. Make associations between what you are learning and something else you have already learned, or rewrite it in your own words or visualise it, so that you absorb the meaning, not just remembering the words.

Chunking is a good example of elaborative rehearsal. Chunking means grouping information in a way that is easy to remember, like breaking the number 462385197 into smaller pieces: 462-385-197. We all come up with tricks to remember numbers. For example, to remember the number 1257 we might think 'the first two numbers are the numbers 1 and 2, so that's easy to remember, and 57 is my house number, so it's the first two counting numbers and my house number'.

The act of rearranging the information or making associations helps us in the elaborative process.

Take a look at the following techniques to make memorisation easier. I recommend that you and your child do this together so you can see your child's reaction to the idea straightaway. Try one technique and then another, and let your child decide which strategies are appealing. When you get stuck, or if something doesn't work, just pick a different one and have another go at the problem. The most important thing is to stay positive and keep trying. All being well, it won't be long before your child is inspired to create his own strategies.

Bite-size chunks

Breaking tasks into bite-sized chunks makes dealing with large amounts of information or a complex problem more manageable. Try and find logical ways to divide the material into smaller parts or sections. Look for ways to group similar information so you can remember it more easily. Look also for associations between what you are learning with what you already know.

Use Post-it notes or a poster board to organise your thoughts, highlight key information, use memory joggers or draw Mind Maps®, to organise information into logical groups. Then work at memorising one section at a time. Concentrate on holding new information in your memory before you move on to the next section. Take a few seconds' break and then return to the first piece of information and try to remember it again. Remember the golden rules of memorisation: practice and repetition.

Mind Mapping®

Tony Buzan[39] is the inventor of a technique he calls Mind Mapping®. He is considered one of today's leading authorities on how the mind works and is the founder of the World Memory Championships. Mind Mapping® is a technique widely used in business and schools, and you can use it at home too.

Mind Mapping® is particularly beneficial for children with dyslexia to help plan essays, organise ideas, solve problems and to summarise revision topics.

Mind Maps® rely on colours, symbols and pictures, rather than using many words, so they are well suited to visual learners who have trouble organising their thoughts using words. You can certainly use words as well, but the dyslexic learner might be more comfortable with just a few words plus images and pictures. (This used to be called a spider diagram.) You draw connecting lines to the images, the same way as you connect ideas in your brain. In this way, you can provide an overall structure using a Mind Map® that makes it easier for someone with dyslexia to see the steps towards the 'big picture', a concept that people with dyslexia often have trouble with when relying on words alone.

To create a Mind Map®, Buzan recommends that you start in the centre of the paper and work outwards.[40] This gives you the greatest freedom to think creatively. Start with a central idea, preferably a picture. Use colours to express different ideas as you move outwards from the centre, capturing other thoughts and ideas that relate to each other. Connect related ideas with lines, and use single keywords to express each one. Buzan also emphasises that you should use curved rather than straight lines to make the Mind Map® visually more interesting and stimulating to your brain.

Using Mind Maps® makes it easier to brainstorm the structure of an essay, the plot of a novel or an outline for a project. It's also a great way to revise for a history exam or even map out the functional relationships of a maths problem. Not only will it help you understand and think about a problem, but you will have a great reference chart at the end of it with all the ideas captured on a single page.

When children with dyslexia read a story and find it difficult to remember the storyline, encourage them to stop and Mind Map® the storyline or draw pictures of what they are reading. Drawing out the story in a visual way helps them see the interrelating parts so that they can develop a picture of the whole story as they read. This technique will take some patience, but it can open up a book in a whole new way to a student with dyslexia, who may even develop a love of reading once he begins to see the plot of the story evolving.

A child with dyslexia will need help learning how to create a Mind Map® – at first, it might seem rather overwhelming – so keep it simple to start with. However, if a child is helped to acquire and build up this skill, the memory benefits are huge.

Mnemonics

This is a highly recommended approach for memorisation and works especially well for remembering lists. It is often used by medical students to learn the muscle groups and bones. Making up mnemonics is easy and you will quickly learn to make up your own. To do so, take the first letter of each word you need to remember and make a new word with each one. It helps if you tie the words together in a sentence. To 'undo' the mnemonic, think of the first letter of each word in the sentence, and then associate it with the word you are trying to remember that starts with that letter.

You will probably remember these music mnemonics from school to remember the lines of treble clef: EGBDF – 'Every Good Boy Deserves Fruit'; and to remember the spaces between the lines: FACE

The fact that you can make up your own sentences makes it fun too, because you can come up with sentences that make you laugh.

Take a look at the following websites for subject-specific mnemonics: **www.mnemonic-device.eu** or **www.eudesign.com/mnems**.

Acronyms

Acronyms are another good way to remember lists of things. Instead of forming a sentence, you take the first letter of each word to make a memorable word. For example, if your child forgets the sequence in which to lay out his work at school, the acronym 'DUMTUMS' can be used: Date, Underline, Miss a line, Title, Underline, Miss a line, Start.

Acronyms are great for remembering biology facts such as the characteristics of a living organism. For example, MR GRINE: **M**ovement, **R**eproduction, **G**rowth, **R**espiration, **I**rritability, **N**utrition, **E**xcretion. Or geography facts such as the famous acronym HOMES to remember the Great Lakes in the United States and Canada: **H**uron, **O**ntario, **M**ichigan, **E**rie and **S**uperior. You still have to learn the names of the lakes but using a memory jogger to think of the first letter makes it easier to recall the unfamiliar-sounding names.

Poems, rhymes and images

Another trick that works well for remembering things is to use a funny rhyme or saying. A famous one I still use helps me remember the number of days in each month:

30 days has September, April, June and November;
All the rest have 31, excepting February alone,
which has but 28 days clear and 29 in each leap year.

Another rhyme that is useful for remembering a spelling rule is:
'i' before 'e' except after 'c'

This is a good way to remember that in words such as 'friend,' 'fiend', 'achieve' and 'grieve', the 'i' comes before the 'e'. But in the word 'receive' the 'e' comes before the 'i' because they follow the letter 'c'.

You can make up your own rhymes, sentences and sayings and come up with silly rhymes that make you laugh. This will also make them easier to remember. Write out the thing you need to remember and then figure out a saying or rhyme to help you remember it. While you are trying to figure it out, subconsciously you will also be creating familiarity with the words and helping to move them from your short-term to your long-term memory. After you have struggled to come up with a trick for remembering, you will find that you may have already automatically remembered some information.

Using peg words

This strategy consists of finding words that rhyme with the words you need to remember. An example is the old English nursery rhyme that teaches counting:

> One, two, tie my shoe
> Three, four, shut the door
> Five, six, pick up sticks
> Seven, eight, lay them straight
> Nine, ten, a big fat hen.

Using peg words often means that you need to learn a new set of words to remember the first set, but it can be easier when you pick your own words. This strategy works best used in conjunction with another strategy such as visualisation. When trying to count to ten in the rhyme above, it is easier to visualise tying your shoes than a one or a two. So, for each peg word, choose a word that allows you to develop a rich mental image.

Remembering numbers

Children often find remembering numbers very difficult, as there is no visual image attached to these unimaginative shapes. By using a rhyming word and pictures, we can associate images with each number. This 'pegging' technique helps children remember a sequence of numbers or number bonds. Get your child to draw images that rhyme with numbers, such as the words below. To remember the number 5824, repeat the rhyme a few times "five eight two four – hive plate shoe door" and visualise/draw the images.

0	1	2	3	4
hero	sun	shoe	tree	door
5	**6**	**7**	**8**	**9**
hive	sticks	heaven	plate	line

Make up a story

When we create acronyms and mnemonics, we are using the first letters of words to form new associations. This is a useful and effective way to learn lists. But what if we want to remember the exact words? Creating a story that uses the words is one way to do this. It will most likely end up being a nonsense story, and that's half the fun. Creating a story from words is a popular game and is a fun pastime on a long car journey, for example. When you make it into a game, you go round the room and everyone adds a piece to the story. When you use it as a learning device, you string the words that you are trying to remember together in a story. Here's an example. Imagine you need to remember some items on a shopping list. The list looks like this:

coffee, sugar, eggs, milk, chicken, tomato soup

We can make the list into a (visualised) short story:

When Anna wakes up she makes a cup of coffee with milk and sugar and then goes out to the barn to gather the eggs that Freda the chicken lays. Then she puts some tomato soup in a bowl with a lid and takes it to work for her lunch.

When you get to the store, visualise the story in your head to remember the items. Incidentally, cutting out pictures from magazine advertisements is another great way to remember grocery items. We return to that later.

Index and flash cards

Using index cards is a great memory tool because you can incorporate several memory strategies at once and will have a handy reference to consult whenever you want to remember something or refresh your memory before a test. Index cards help you to break information into manageable pieces.

You can cut pictures from magazines, use coloured markers to create your own pictures and memory joggers, and rearrange the index cards to play with grouping the information until you find the way that is easiest for you to remember. You can store the cards so that you can review them later. Use envelopes to sort cards for different subjects and store them in a special box so that you won't have to search for them later.

Read the cards several times, taking time between each card to focus on the information. For very important information or an exam, read the cards over at night before you go to bed, and then again in the morning when you get up.

Flash cards (like blank playing cards) are smaller than index cards and are great for remembering small amounts of information such as times tables, spellings and phonic sounds.

Say it out loud

Use this strategy alone or in conjunction with the index card strategy. Read a passage to yourself silently and then test yourself to see how much you remember. Read the next passage out loud and see if you remember more. When we read out loud we are using the simple principle of employing more senses at once.

Typically, when we read out loud, we read more slowly than when we read silently in our minds. In silent reading, we often skip the unimportant words. It's the difference between getting the general gist of something and really understanding the full meaning. Because short-term memory does not hold very much information – sometimes only one or two seconds'-worth for some people – saying something out loud, more slowly means that the information goes into your memory in smaller amounts, so is easier to remember.

Summarise

When you read something significant that you want to remember, stop and summarise it in one sentence (out loud or in your head). Knowing in your mind that you are going to have to summarise or remember out loud what you have just read forces the mind subconsciously to pay more attention.

This strategy is even more effective if you make a note or two, or write an index card as a memory jogger. If you are reading something complex, consider making a Mind Map® or poster as you go. This not only helps you to remember but also tests your understanding. What's more, you will end up with some reference materials that you can return to so that you reinforce learning by studying again later on.

DIVA

In my experience, I have found it is important to use stimulating approaches that talk to a child's imagination in any subject. I believe teaching methods should be creative and include:

- **D**ramatisation
- **I**magination
- **V**isualisation
- **A**ssociation

Dramatisation

Dramatisation is a fun way of memorising key sequences, facts or stories. It is not about memorising large quantities of text or information verbatim but is considered to be a bodily kinaesthetic version of association (see below). It is a way of making information or learning material more memorable.

Verbal and/or visual spatial abilities in children with dyslexia are often their best strength. So is empathy. Through role play, freeze frame or drama activities, children develop empathy and acquire a deeper understanding of characters, plot, theme and atmosphere of studied literature, historical events, religious studies and so forth.

Some children enjoy this method of memorising facts, as they are in less danger of experiencing failure.

Imagination

Children with dyslexia often have rich imaginations and many great ideas. Tapping into children's imaginations at any age makes learning fun. Even if children don't enjoy reading, they love listening to stories and telling their own story. Stories and hands-on activities can stimulate their imagination, help put learning into context and help children remember what they are learning.

Often, children's difficulty comes from getting their many wonderful and wild ideas down on paper and in the right order. We can help them direct their imagination skills through brainstorming, using games and pictures and writing templates to help stimulate and focus their ideas into logical sequences.

Visualisation

Children with dyslexia often have great creative ability. Visuals such as pictures, charts and diagrams are especially useful, but you can also create pictures and moving images in your head. Making associations and visual reference points are key strategies in remembering. We do it to some degree subconsciously. Make the process fun by coming up with funny images to remember things by.

Here are some ideas to pass on to your child or teenager.

- Use visualisation as children read a passage that is new to them and to help them remember the content of a comprehension exercise or poem. Encourage them to create a picture in their mind that is easy to remember, and take a pretend photo or video doing all the actions, which will make it come alive. Then, press the 'replay button' to practise over and over.

- Visualisation is a good way to remember your way round the school building or to a friend's house. As you walk, notice things around you and associate landmarks with where you are going. Perhaps you glimpse a poster through a classroom window and you know this is where you need to turn, or maybe there is a light on one side of the hallway where you need to turn and not on the other. When you are walking to your friend's house, perhaps you notice a red front door where you have to turn and then you notice a post box at the next place you need to turn.

- When you have bulleted lists of text, use a marker to add a coloured dot next to the important points. Use different colours for different ideas: green can be dates, red can be facts of historical significance and blue can be ideas or opinions – you get the idea.

- For remembering numbers, for example, visualise the number one is always an orange square, the number two is always a green circle etc. After using the same technique for a while, it will be familiar and easy to do.

Over time, children can develop some consistent tricks for remembering things. There are more tips in the **Literacy skills** chapter.

Association

You can use association to develop a technique for associating a new fact with an old one – or associating it with a picture or image in your mind. When you recall the old information, it will also be easier to remember the new information. This builds on the ideas we talked about earlier, where information from long-term memory is called into the working memory to process new information. Association brings this memory operation to a conscious level, and allows you to focus more easily on new, unfamiliar information.

One technique for applying association is called 'chaining' or linking. This is used for remembering a list of random things in the exact order in which you wish to recall them.

The essence of the system is to create a mental picture of two adjacent items in the list that links them memorably. This is most likely if the picture or image is vivid and unusual and incorporates genuine interaction, so you create a story where one idea leads to the next. It is a useful technique for learning lists of random items or facts. For example: imagine you have to remember the words lamp, book and computer. You make up a story using those words in the order you want to remember them.

The loci memory system

'Loci' is the Latin word for 'places'. This memory system basically depends on the mental association of remembering what you heard or saw when you were in a particular place. For example, you might be talking to a friend when a big red bus passes you in the high street.

When you recall the image of the bus, you can also recall the conversation you had with your friend. Some people use this method to visualise walking along a path that has distinctive landmarks. Link each landmark in your mind to what you want to remember. Then, whenever you take your visual walk and pass the landmarks, you can remember the things you associated with them.

Study buddy

One of the most effective and fun ways to learn is to teach someone else. Having a study buddy or studying in a group enables you to ask questions, explain your understanding and learn from your peers. You are more likely to remember things when you have group interaction because you will be making subconscious associations between your interactions with the group and your learning. It is always interesting to hear another person's perspective and their techniques for remembering. We all think in different ways and hearing someone else's take on something can help us see it in a new light.

Test yourself

After you read a passage or a list of words that you need to remember, stop to ask yourself questions, or try to recall the list. Note down how much you remember. Read the passage or list again and repeat the exercise.

Repetition, repetition, repetition

Playing games

Games are a great way to relieve stress, have fun, enjoy a break and practise good memory skills at the same time. You can find many good games in shops and on the Internet – but you can easily make them up using common household items and a little imagination. Playing games regularly really helps to strengthen your memory muscles. Depending on how competitive you feel, you need not think of the games as having a winner or a loser. Play them for fun until you tire of them. Here are some ideas for memory games.

I went to market

You could play this game (with at least one other person) to remember Spanish vocabulary words. One person starts out with the first sentence: 'I went to market and I bought 'una naranja' (an orange). The next person repeats that and adds to the list, then you have to repeat both the first item and the new item, and add another, so: 'I went to market and I bought a 'una naranja', y 'un plátano' (a banana). The game continues in this way until one of you cannot repeat the list any longer or both of you fall about laughing.

Simon says

Use a variation of the old favourite, 'Simon says'. In the traditional game, one person stands at the front and gives an instruction, 'Simon says, touch your (nose). The others have to do what Simon says. In the memory version, you add more instructions. So, for example learning Spanish vocabulary 'Simon says, touch your 'nariz' (nose) with your finger and then rub your 'estómago' (tummy). And, 'Simon says, touch your 'nariz', rub your 'estómago' and stomp 'un pie' (a foot). Keep building the list until the players cannot keep up with you any longer.

The tray game (Kim's game)

This is the game where you place items on a tray, hold it out for about ten seconds and then remove the tray. But try this variation. Put only three items on the tray to start. The other player has to remember the three items. Then remove the tray and add a fourth item. Bring the tray back for ten seconds and have the other player remember all the items. Keep building the number of items on the tray until the other player can no longer remember them all.

Not all these tips, tricks and strategies will work for everyone. Select the techniques or tips that you think may work for your child. If they do not work, review the list and try something else. Eventually, your child will develop his own list of strategies and techniques that work best for him.

Technology memory tools

Technology is especially useful for dyslexic learners and, if you can afford to equip your child with some electronic gadgets, they can help to alleviate some common problems. Some of the most frustrating difficulties for people with dyslexia, such as forgetting appointments, phone numbers and addresses, can be overcome by today's technology tools.

Mobile phones are obviously great for storing phone numbers, and many have the ability to store voice recordings, as well as make written text notes, which can all be emailed and included in documents. The calendar function is useful for setting different alarm tones for different appointments.

Computers, laptops, notebooks, iPads, Kindles or handheld PDAs (Personal Digital Assistant) have revolutionised learning for children with dyslexia. They are not only useful for recording and storing information, but are indispensable for checking phonetic spelling errors, grammar, punctuation, text to speech and speech to text. iPhones and iPads are invaluable for downloading free apps (applications) such as dictionaries, times tables, spellings, educational podcasts, children's reading books, memory games and much more.

Microsoft Outlook® is very useful, providing several different visual views, and can run on a lightweight PDA to monitor appointments, store contact information for friends, family and teachers, and keep track of homework tasks, revision schedules and due dates easily.

There are also many assistive technology programmes to choose from that allow you to generate memory aids, create graphics, charts, presentations and other visual materials and many that have speech to text facilities. Those dyslexic learners who have trouble sitting still to read and write are more at home with the interactive nature of tapping on a keyboard, pointing and clicking with the mouse and using interactive software to master a variety of subjects.

Technology is extremely helpful in acquiring and practising memory skills in a fun and motivating way, but not to the exclusion of manual, traditional methods. In the **Appendix**, you can find suppliers of special educational needs resources.

Global positioning system (GPS)

For your older child who is learning to drive, map reading or remembering directions may prove to be confusing. In addition to the GPS devices used for driving that have spoken directions and maps, there is a wide variety of handheld devices that are useful for navigating short distances. They can be used by children who like to go places on foot but who sometimes forget the route. Using GPS on mobile phones or watches, they can set waypoints as well as start and end points, in order to navigate their route more easily.

Other electronic devices

Depending on what your child needs help with, there are several different types of lightweight portable devices that can assist your child.

There is a wide variety of smart phones that act as a calendar, a notebook, an alarm clock, an address book, reminders, and so on. The alarm setting on a digital watch can be used for lesson reminders and may be more reliable than mobile phones which may run out of battery. Voice recorders can be used to make voice notes for homework, appointments, travel directions, etc.

Technology is always improving and getting smaller, more portable and less expensive, so keep your eye on the latest developments and make use of new devices as they come along.

A word of caution when your child uses technology; watch out for any of the health problems surrounding excessive use of tablet devices, computer screens and eReader technology. Known side effects include eye strain, headaches, dizziness, nausea, unfocused attention, laziness, insomnia, muscle aches and even depression, obesity or technology addiction. It's best not to use technology at least two hours before bedtime.

A holistic approach to memory

A holistic approach to raising children that focuses on the body, spirit and mind works particularly well with children who have dyslexia. A holistic approach is just as important for the good functioning of memory. If your child is hungry or tired, he is less likely to study well and his memory will not perform at its best. If he is worried or stressed, his heart will not be open to learning, and he will not perform well.

Distractions, even little ones, are hard for children to resist. It takes a lifetime to learn to tune things out, shut the door on noise, switch off mobile phones, stop checking our emails, turn off the TV or whatever else helps us concentrate better. The world of studying, which mostly involves reading and writing, is a difficult one for people with dyslexia, and a child who is still learning to develop discipline and good study habits is vulnerable to every distraction.

A child's emotional state is very important when learning and trying to remember new information. His memory performance can also be affected by how motivated he is and the intensity of an experience. When an experience inspires a strong emotion in us because it is unusual, exciting, scary, sad, and so on, it is much easier to remember. Likewise, if learning is fun and exciting, our hearts are more open to the learning experience, and we are more likely to make a connection and remember the information. It is also easier to remember information about something we are interested in.

A child's emotional state is very important when learning new information

Help your child to set up a peaceful, comfortable working environment, eat nutritious food at regular intervals, and get to bed on time. A regular routine and a cosy study area will go a long way in helping your child find his focus and apply his concentration for the best possible memory results. There is more information in the **Study skills and homework** chapter.

PART THREE
Your Child's Holistic Needs

Chapter 8
Emotional intelligence, self-confidence and self-esteem

The biggest problem with dyslexic kids is not the perceptual problem; it is their perception of themselves. That was my biggest problem.

Bruce Jenner, Olympic athlete[41]

Dyslexia is the result of physical differences in the way our brain works. When people feel 'different', they often experience stress and frustration, which can lead to negative emotions. Low self-esteem, anxiety and depression can accompany feelings of deep frustration, anger and fear. Negative emotions affect the way our brain functions, making us unable to think clearly or rationally. When we are in an emotional state or inner turmoil, it is difficult to get into a learning state of mind, because we feel unsafe and fearful. We go into fight or flight mode and the amygdala (in the brain) kicks in to protect the body and mind. Emotions and self-esteem play a massive role in enabling our children to learn effectively.

The good news is that some great strides have been made recently in the field of emotional intelligence (EI). The term refers to our ability to recognise, understand and manage our emotions and those of others.

When learning is addressed from a holistic perspective, addressing emotional as well as academic issues, the child with dyslexia does much better overall, often learning to accommodate dyslexia without negative feelings.

John Gottman is a well-known psychologist who has spent many years studying family dynamics. In his book, *Raising an*

Emotionally Intelligent Child: The Heart of Parenting (1998), he emphasises how parenting can make a tremendous difference to a child's self-esteem and level of emotional intelligence. He describes two types of parents: those who fail to teach children how to deal with their emotions and those who practise what he calls 'Emotion-Coaching'. The latter raise children who are better at controlling their emotional state and suffer less frustration and, interestingly, fewer illnesses than other children. Emotionally coached students are also better on the whole at focusing on academic studies, and do better in school.

Emotionally coached students are also better on the whole at focusing on academic studies, and do better in school

According to Dr Gottman, an important parenting skill is becoming aware of your child's emotional state. We need to learn how to help children deal with negative feelings, including stress, frustration, anger and depression. He recommends that, when we detect strong emotions in our child, we use this as an opportunity to teach him how to handle the emotion. This includes, above all, acknowledging and validating the feeling, and then helping him find words to express it. We can then move on to explore strategies with our child for coping with the emotion and diffusing rather than suppressing it.

Emotional intelligence (EI)

The field of emotional intelligence is relatively new and has evolved rapidly since the 1990s. EI is how you understand yourself and others. I believe that EI is a significant precursor to a healthy mind, body and soul.

With recent advances in educational thinking, it is becoming widely accepted that an IQ test measures only certain intelligence areas, and people who do poorly in these traditionally measured areas may well excel in other areas that are not tested in the same way. Therefore, an IQ test is not sufficient to measure a person's *whole* intelligence. That is why, during an assessment, it is important also to use observation techniques and find out what else the child is good at (that tests can't do) to gain a greater holistic understanding of a child's overall abilities.

Emotional intelligence is another form of intelligence or maturity that a person experiences or manifests. Researchers agree that EI is an important factor in how we operate and interact in society and forms a component of our overall intelligence.

In 1995, Daniel Goleman published a book called *Emotional Intelligence* that has had a big influence on the way we think of this area. In his book, Goleman outlines five domains of emotional intelligence:[42]

- Knowing your emotions
- Managing your own emotions
- Motivating yourself
- Recognising and understanding other people's emotions
- Managing relationships, i.e., managing the emotions of others.

Emotional intelligence is an important part of developing into a well-rounded adult. People with dyslexia need to be very self-aware. Later on I talk about metacognition – the ability to be aware of your own learning style in order to help yourself learn more easily. Like other intelligences, it can be practised and acquired through teaching children people skills: communication, cooperation, resolving conflict, managing emotions, empathy and self-awareness. Mastery of emotional intelligence is an excellent skill for people with dyslexia.

Traditionally, schools and the workplace have discouraged the idea of showing emotion. We frown upon those who are prone to emotional outbursts. Consequently, we learn to suppress those feelings in public and reserve our outbursts for the privacy of our own home. Emotional intelligence is the study of how emotions are inevitably tied to everything we do. Suppressing our feelings is not the same as learning to manage them. Just as we can learn to tie our shoes, read a book and perform complex mathematical computations, we can learn to study and even anticipate our emotions and to recognise and manage triggers that set off deep feelings and knee-jerk reactions.

Not only should we learn to control our emotions, but schools can also adapt to accommodate emotional aspects of learning. Teachers can teach around our emotions, offering support and addressing issues that are likely to trigger us. One example is maths anxiety: deep emotions are often associated with problems in maths. For dyslexic learners, similar anxiety can be associated with reading, spelling and writing. Adapting teaching methods to address anxiety can free children from stress and enable them to focus on learning.

Fight or flight response

At the root of our emotional framework, the limbic system (the emotional brain) is responsible for emotions, pleasure, behaviour, motivation and emotional association with memory. The amygdala is recognised as the mechanism that controls or calls upon these emotions.

The amygdala is deeply connected with our 'fight or flight' response in the face of unexpected stress and is a primitive, necessary reaction for survival. The amygdala reacts very quickly, much more quickly than the cognitive processing areas of the brain. We can understand this better by considering a specific situation. Let's use the maths anxiety problem again. When a child who has trouble with maths is called on in class to go to the board and solve a problem, the fight or flight response happens much more quickly than the child's cognitive processing. Perhaps the maths problem is not that difficult; but the amygdala has already sent out its signals to the brain and fear sets in.

When stress kicks in, the amygdala triggers a lightning-fast response, sometimes called 'emotional hijacking', as it hijacks our rational brain and is taken over by an emotional reaction that prevents us from thinking clearly and logically.

In this highly emotional state, our brain will react by kicking in with one of two reactions: fight or flight. In fight mode, you react to the situation by confronting it head on. In flight mode, you seek to escape from the situation as quickly as possible.

Various emotions are associated with each state. By observing your child in various stressful situations you can learn to identify which mode he is in. Here are some common manifestations:

- Fight responses: shouting; bad behaviour; becoming abusive; becoming threatening; lashing out
- Flight responses: withdrawal; tuning out; shutting down; going blank; crying; freezing; avoiding

Being in fight or flight mode affects our bodies in many ways. Our heart speeds up, our lungs work harder, our body may shake, our digestion slows down, our bowel becomes tense, our bladder relaxes, our vision and hearing may become distorted and our reflexes most certainly speed up. But children and teenagers do not understand these physical or emotional reactions to fear, danger or anticipated pain.

When you recognise the fight or flight reaction in your young child or teenager, allow him time to calm down. It may take a few minutes or hours to overcome the reaction. This is a good time to take a break. Let your child de-stress by chilling out, or better still, playing or running outside to use up the adrenalin that rushes in when the fight or flight response is in full swing.

The fight or flight response hits us all, parents and children alike. You can probably relate to similar feelings when your child does something you don't approve of. Think of how you feel when you learn that your child has forgotten his homework for the fourth time that week or that he has done something you have expressly asked him not to do. Do you feel anger rise up? What about when you realise he is late coming home from school, it's dark outside, and you have no idea where he is? Do you feel a sudden rush of fear?

It is important to understand that parents too can be emotionally hijacked by the amygdala. By paying attention to our feelings and sudden rush of negative emotions, we can learn to control fight or flight symptoms. When you recognise this response in your child, wait before administering punishment. Give yourself time out and allow the logical processing of the brain to kick back in before you respond.

People react to fear in different ways. Some shut down while others get angry. The reaction depends in part on our personality and in part on the physical reaction in our brain. Once fear has set in, it consumes our mental focus and takes over our working memory so that we are unable to focus on the problem at hand, which affects our ability to learn. Knowing that this physical reaction takes place when a child with dyslexia is called on to read out loud or give a presentation allows us to rethink the teaching method. Our emotions are inextricably linked with learning, which means that schools need to be involved in emotional development.

Anxiety is an expression of fear: the fear of being inadequate and the fear of failure when faced with situations that are new or complicated. Dyslexic learners need time to process information and get used to new situations. For example, if a class changes location and a child has suddenly to find a new classroom, this can create anxiety that is just as deep as the pressure of reading out loud. A common reaction to anxiety is to avoid the situation that causes fear. Teachers and parents may confuse this avoidance with laziness. If a child is skipping class or avoiding doing homework, try to find out why a subject is causing so much fear and anxiety.

Frustration and fear often lead to anger. Children may express their anger at school or at home. Often, a child feels safer at home and therefore lets out more emotion. If you have a very angry child, or your child is prone to angry outbursts, root out the sources of fear and frustration that are provoking the anger. Dealing with an angry child can be intimidating. We feel helpless and don't know what to do because every move is likely to provoke an outburst. However, to help our child, we need to persevere and find a way to help him deal with the source of the anger.

Our emotional state or mood also affects what we remember. We remember emotionally-charged events more easily than boring ones (the Von Restorff effect). When we are depressed, we remember negative things and when we are happy, we remember positive things. The stronger the emotions aroused, the more likely we are to remember something.

Our attention span also seems to be associated with our emotional state. When we are emotionally aroused, a state of activity is triggered in our brains that either distracts us (such as when we become angry while we are driving) or helps us to focus. This state of activity is an automatic response that sets us on guard so we are ready to respond to a situation – the fight or flight state.

What fight or flight means to parents

Behaviour in children can be influenced through emotional intelligence awareness and education. Seattle Children's Hospital Research Foundation Patient and Family Education Division published a booklet entitled *Problem Solving With Your Child*, in which the authors explore the parent–child relationship with respect to emotional intelligence and talk about recognising your child's cognitive and maturity levels, and his emotional intelligence level.

When your child gets angry and you recognise the anger is caused by the fight reaction triggered by the amygdala, and is not just bad behaviour, you can respond quite differently. When parents understand a child's emotional intelligence and adapt their parenting style accordingly, children are less likely to experience behaviour problems.

When we are in the grip of emotional reactions, it is harder for us to help our children develop their own emotional intelligence. As we become more emotionally aware, it is easier to help our children develop their emotions.

Self-confidence and self-esteem

I have talked about what dyslexia is and the manifestations that are symptomatic or indicative of the condition in children. I also talk about the wonderful and positive attributes that can be the result of dyslexia and the many talents that children with dyslexia can have. But how does this relate to your child?

Self-confidence is the degree to which we believe in our abilities (what we can do), and self-esteem is about valuing ourselves as people and feeling we are good enough (how we regard ourselves).

Self-confidence and self-esteem feed upon each other: low self-esteem will lead to lack of confidence in our ability and vice versa.

Children start to compare themselves to their peers from a very early age. From the moment your child begins to find school work difficult, or finds out he has dyslexia, he is up against one of his biggest challenges, that of feeling he is somehow different from others in the class. Your child's self-confidence at the point of diagnosis is likely to be at a low ebb and probably played a big part in your decision to have your child assessed.

Diagnosis can seem like a good and a bad thing. Knowing what you are up against, you can now begin to deal with the finer emotional aspects of dyslexia in positive and constructive ways. There is no denying that there are challenges ahead that may affect your child's self-confidence and self-esteem.

We pay our children compliments, try to boost their ego, tell them how great and how talented they are. But inside, while all children appreciate being loved, they can have a tendency to think, 'Mum/Dad is just saying that because they love me'; and may continue to feel self-doubt. We sense that our words of encouragement do not have the desired effect, and our child's self-esteem remains low.

A lack of self-esteem can get worse as a child moves from primary to secondary (high) school and reaches the age where hormones kick in. Children aged 11–16 can be exceptionally self-conscious about their physical and mental shortcomings. They see themselves as caricatures with all their worst points emphasised. A small spot on the end of their nose or a bad haircut causes them to run into their room and bolt the door.

Peer pressure is another strong force at this age. Children in secondary school have a tendency to break into groups, as they experiment with finding their place in the world. The groups change with each generation, but invariably they form, and invariably teenagers try to fit into one or other of them.

Those who hang around on the periphery and don't fit in to any of the groups are usually loners, or somehow different from other kids. They might be on the eccentric side and unkindly dubbed as 'nerds'. They may not be able to afford the latest trends or gadgets that provide them with common ground in the group; or they might be kids whose parents buy them everything they want at the drop of a hat. They might just be quiet and shy.

It is probably fair to say that most children who don't fit into a group experience feelings of loneliness or of being outsiders. These feelings are not unique to children with dyslexia. Puberty is not selective. We all have to pass through it on our way to growing up. It can be a fine art determining if what your child goes through at any stage of his life is attributable to 'normal' forces or to dyslexia.

> **From the moment your child begins to find school work difficult, or finds out he has dyslexia, he is up against one of his biggest challenges**

From this point forward there are many things you can do to boost your child's self-confidence and self-esteem. Providing your child with coping strategies prepares and sets him up for success.

Developing self-confidence

Children with dyslexia may start out in life full of self-confidence. As they progress through the school system, especially once they realise they are not reading and writing at the same level as their peers, their self-confidence can quickly erode, which leads to feelings of low self-esteem. One of the most important things you can do to help raise his level of self-confidence is to help your child find the things he is good at. When we know we are good at something, it is easier to accept we are not so good at something else.

Find out the things your child is good at

The one thing that can help your child develop his self-confidence is the ability to accomplish things on his own. Initially, he will benefit from much support and continual praise for the slightest accomplishment. Once he has built up his self-confidence, then let him attempt things on his own. You can direct your energy towards helping your child establish routines and strategies for tackling problems resulting from the dyslexia and empowering him to overcome it.

Then comes the hardest part of being a parent: you have to sit back and watch him wrestle with it until he figures out for himself how to deal with it. Only from coping, overcoming and triumphing under their own steam will children's self-esteem truly begin to build up.

**Once they have found their confidence,
nothing will stop them**

How to Raise Self-confidence

- Ask your child to list all his strengths (you may need to remind him what he is good at)
- Encourage your child to focus on his strengths at all times
- Encourage him to have a positive mental attitude
- Set an example of a positive attitude when you are faced with challenges
- Encourage him to try new challenges, develop his talents and set goals
- Teach him to walk 'tall' and smile
- Help him define the area that is causing him to have a lack of self-confidence
- Help him develop the missing skills
- Take plenty of time to practise the missing skills
- Get him to acknowledge his progress and achievement in the problem area
- Give tons of positive reinforcement
- Reassure him that it's OK to make mistakes – that's how we all learn
- Remind your child that you don't have to be perfect to be confident
- Remind him to compliment others: what goes around, comes around
- Remind him to be himself: he is the best, and he is unique

Once children have found their confidence, nothing will stop them. But you cannot find it for them. You can only enable them to find it for themselves.

Developing high self-esteem

High or low self-esteem is the extent to which we appreciate our talents and personality, in short, how much we like ourselves. People with dyslexia who feel they are failing often see themselves as 'stupid' or suffer other people telling them they are silly or lazy. Sometimes, when they succeed, people with dyslexia attribute their success to luck, because success feels unusual, and they fail to translate their success into feelings of high self-esteem.

High self-esteem is vital
to developing into our best self

Not all children with low self-esteem will come across as shy, timid or introverted. Some children become loud, clown-like or extrovert to try to compensate for feelings of inadequacy, lack of friends, workload pressure or problems at home. You need to play detective and watch out for any changes in their behaviour or attitude.

High self-esteem is vital to developing into our best self. The sooner your child is able to talk about his feelings, the sooner he will feel he is not alone and start to feel better about himself.

There is much we can do as parents and educators to help children through the stages of accepting having dyslexia and on to achieving higher self-esteem. We can teach them to be good role models by showing them how to be self-aware and aware of others by:

- respecting themselves
- respecting others
- being responsible for their actions
- focusing on their strengths
- learning how to attempt new tasks and experiences

- being proud of what they achieve
- learning to handle positive and negative emotions

If you have concerns about your child's mental well-being, and you notice his self-esteem is very low or he is self-harming, seek advice from your doctor immediately. It is important to talk to the school and check if staff have noticed a change in your child's behaviour, friendship dynamics or work output, and make sure you all work together.

Techniques to manage low self-esteem

Dyslexia's greatest difficulty is low self-esteem. Children begin school full of curiosity and eagerness to learn, but can quickly become disillusioned by unexpected failure in the classroom. If they are not well-supported through their difficulties at school or their issues are not addressed correctly or quickly, low self-esteem will surely set in. This can lead to alienation and withdrawal, anti-social behaviour, and in extreme cases lead to drug use and self-harm.

Dyslexia's greatest difficulty is low self-esteem

Living in a state of continued frustration, anger and low self-esteem can lead to feelings of depression. Depression can lead to suicidal thoughts and complicates our ability to live happy lives. With the right emotional support and early intervention, children can become happy, healthy individuals.

Signs of depression in children are different from those in adults. Depression can cause children to act up, act violently or generally misbehave. They can typically have a very negative self-image and seem to have difficulty enjoying even life's pleasurable moments. They often do not look forward to the future and have few positive moments or memories.

Sometimes children with low self-esteem behave badly, generally because they are unable to manage their emotions. So we have to balance our levels of diplomacy and tolerance against what is acceptable or unacceptable behaviour and need to set limits on poor behaviour.

We need to create a safe place for our child to express his feelings. Managing self-esteem involves putting our feelings into a language that we can articulate and understand. Our aim when raising self-esteem is to help our children feel good about themselves and steer them in a more positive direction.

Here are some tips to get your child talking:

- Choose your moment and remain calm
- Don't wait for a meltdown or tantrum
- Listen and be understanding and supportive
- Get to the bottom of the problem or feeling
- Acknowledge the problem
- Help your child break down big problems into smaller, manageable ones
- Emphasise positive aspects of your child's performance or behaviour
- Draw on past successes
- Agree an action plan with your child
- Monitor progress against the plan

Once a child is able to express and understand his problem and emotions and feels that you understand too, you can start putting a healing plan into action.

Helping young children express their emotions

Telling stories and sharing our story is great emotional therapy and helps communicate and develop good relationships. Personal stories are a way to impart advice and information about something we have struggled with or triumphed over, and help us assimilate and learn from our own experiences. By speaking them out loud and reliving them through our own recounting, we etch them in our memories and store their lessons for future use.

We relay our story to comfort each other and create a feeling of empathy or bonding with others going through similar experiences, both good and bad. It's good to know that we are not the only ones, that others have had to deal with similar situations, and that they lived to see another day.

It should come as no surprise that storytelling and role play are used in a therapeutic way to help children with learning challenges.[43] Stories using the third person are a simple, non-threatening way to teach your child how to deal with a multitude of difficulties, including how to express and control anger and frustration, and how to cope with being teased at school.

To make the story appealing and to captivate younger listeners, try using cute animals, for example, as protagonists in your story. You could create a simple story about a baby rabbit that has trouble reading and is laughed at in class by the other rabbits. Mummy rabbit offers advice and comfort, and practises reading with the baby rabbit at home. Baby rabbit learns to read a few new words, and in class the next day is praised by his teacher.

You can invent stories about anything. Keep them simple and short and your child will enjoy listening to them, while the power of the message gives him tools to cope. There is also great suggestive power in the story of a magic charm, such as a stone or a special object that the hero carries around in a pocket. He touches the stone whenever he feels bad, and it helps him feel better and accomplish a difficult task. Keep the story slightly distant from the real problem, changing it so that you don't touch a nerve. It's important to choose the right time of day and make sure your child is cosy and comfortable before you begin.

Diane Haugen, in her article *Telling History*,[44] reminds us that the human brain has an outstanding capacity for pattern recognition and that stories get filed away in our memory to provide pattern templates on which we can then draw to compare with our personal experience.

If a child listens to positive stories about problem solving in general, even if he is not currently experiencing a particular problem, he will have plenty of memories to draw on when similar problems surface. This is the theory behind the telling of fairy tales, where good generally triumphs over evil. After listening to a wealth of fairy tales and fables, young children have plenty of examples of good and evil with which to compare real-life situations, as they process childhood experiences on their way to adulthood.

Stories are also useful the other way round, when your child helps to create them. Allow an eager child to give you inputs to the story, or even make up his own story, but don't force it. Perhaps he would find comfort in listening rather than talking. When you invite your child to help you develop the plot in a story, you will find out what is bothering him and what problems he is working on in his mind. Sometimes children experience a depth of feeling that they have trouble recognising, and they have difficulty giving names to particular emotions. They cannot always express what is bothering them, and therefore behave badly for reasons we do not always understand.

As children get older, they will, ideally, learn to articulate these thoughts and feelings, but young children have trouble even understanding that something *is* bothering them. They feel out of sorts and cannot explain it to you. Psychologists often use role play with puppets or dolls and, by observing their play, can get insights into what is going on in the child's life.

Helping older children express themselves

While storytelling works well with younger children, older children need to express themselves in more mature ways. As they grow up, analogies can work well to help them get their feelings out. For example, a volcano can be a metaphor for the way in which difficult feelings such as frustration, hurt and injustice can build up inside us over time. When we suppress feelings, pressure accumulates to the point that even a minor annoyance can easily trigger an adolescent (as well as an adult) to 'blow his top'.

You can think of other analogies that teens can relate to, or let them think up their own. Vivid dreams and nightmares can also be indicative of emotional turmoil. At this age, teenagers start to remember their dreams and ponder their meaning deeply. For example, dreams about falling or sliding in a car with no brakes, or being unable to stop a car hurtling at full speed are indicative of feeling out of control. If your teenager wants to discuss a dream, encourage him to remember as much about it as possible. Remembering will help him sort it out on a conscious or unconscious level. If a dream seems particularly turbulent, ask what is bothering him and help him figure out ways to deal with it.

Therapies to manage low self-esteem

If children refuse to communicate with parents, there are several other techniques or therapies you can investigate to help manage their emotions. More and more families are seeking alternative therapy for their children as a means to reduce stress, improve behaviour and find ways to make their children feel physically and mentally good about themselves. Therapies such as acupuncture, massage, cranio-sacral massage, reflexology, homeopathy, Neuro-linguistic Programming (NLP), Emotional Freedom Technique (EFT), Mindfulness-based Cognitive Therapy (MBCT), spiritual healing, yoga and listening therapies can be uplifting ways to raise self-esteem, relax or reduce symptoms of anxiety, stress or depression. Art therapy, play therapy and music therapy all have their place in helping children deal with their emotions.

Having alternative therapy is a very personal choice, with which you may or may not feel comfortable – but try to keep an open mind. Alternative therapies that do not involve using drugs should be investigated. A high percentage of families with ADHD children seek alternative therapies, rather than resorting to drugs. These therapies are good for the whole family. If your child is stressed out, you might be too. Some schools are even introducing Mindfulness in school to help students relax, stop worrying and focus on the here and now.

Here is more information on some of the therapies I have mentioned:

Neuro-linguistic programming (NLP)

Neuro-linguistic programming is a technique to help children or adults learn to break down negative patterns, thoughts and emotions, in order to be able to respond more positively. It is used in business, life and education to help individuals build self-confidence, overcome anxiety or phobias and improve communication skills.

NLP works by helping us adapt our ways of thinking, feeling and behaving to certain situations and can help children learn to believe in themselves and deal with situations more successfully. NLP workshops are a fun way to build up self-esteem and confidence levels by using games, activities, practical exercises and role play.

Emotional freedom technique (EFT) and tapping for kids

The Emotional Freedom Technique is a way to channel energy and emotion in the body to enhance psychological health and well-being. 'Tapping' is an activity that involves tapping on various pressure points on the body – similar to acupressure. Along with the physical tapping, it uses stories and rhyme to show children how to use EFT to express and defuse their emotions.

The tapping technique for children is attributed to Australian EFT practitioner Angie Muccillo, who has written *Tapping for Kids: A Children's Guide to Emotional Freedom Technique* (2008). In Muccillo's book, using the technique, children metaphorically enter a palace that they explore one floor at a time, beginning with the playshop on the ground floor. Here they find out about the body's energy system. As they progress through the palace, they learn how to call up inner powers and explore their feelings. As they discover feelings such as anger and sadness, they learn how to deal with them. At the top of the palace, on the eighth floor, is the graduation room. Along the way, they learn how to use a feeling meter, with which they can assess what they are feeling and monitor their own progress. They can also make up their own stories, songs and poems.

Tapping has been shown to provide considerable help and comfort to children working through strong emotions, especially feelings of fear and dread, anger and depression. It requires an adult to teach the child how to do it and works best if the counsellor has some background in EFT. Talk to your school counsellors and find out their level of knowledge or expertise in the approach or see if they can recommend you to a trained

EFT specialist. Once children have learned to tap, they can use the technique on their own. It provides children with the freedom to control their emotional state and calm down or empower themselves when they feel anxious or overwhelmed.

Mindfulness-based cognitive therapy (MBCT)

MBCT is delivered by qualified counsellors or psychologists. It is used to help children or adults deal with anxiety, depression, bullying, OCD, eating disorders, low self-esteem and behavioural problems. MBCT is goal oriented, placing emphasis on the role that thoughts play with regard to emotions and behaviours. MBCT is based on the concept that thoughts and reactions are learned, rather than inbuilt, and can be unlearned and replaced with positive, empowering thoughts. The therapist generally needs to work with both parent and child when the child is young. Different therapists suggest different minimum ages for children to have MBCT. Children need sufficient cognitive skills to engage actively but, as a guideline, around 8 years onwards is likely.

If you suspect that your child is depressed, he will be in pain and needs help. I urge you to seek professional help and not to wait for the problem to get better by itself. Talk to your school counsellor to discuss solutions at school and visit your family doctor or a child psychologist/therapist.

Children need an outlet to release their feelings of frustration and inadequacy brought about by having dyslexia or any learning difference. If we focus on helping our children manage their emotions and build up their levels of self-confidence, it is more likely that they will develop higher levels of self-esteem. If we lead by example and understand and manage our own feelings and frustrations well, we are more likely to be able to help our children manage theirs. Positive self-esteem is fundamental to our mental well-being: it is fundamental for building healthy relationships with others and also helps us handle new situations better.

Chapter 9
Road to your child's success – part I: body, mind and soul

My friends have always known I've had a bit
of trouble with spelling and reading and I
think having that support and
encouragement is the most important aspect
of being dyslexic.

Kara Tointon, actress[45]

If you do not have dyslexia yourself, it can be difficult to understand what your child is thinking and feeling. You are up against all the usual aspects of raising a child, a challenge for the best of us at the best of times, with the added challenge of trying to understand and help your child work with his dyslexia.

Where do the 'usual' problems end and the special ones begin? How much of your child's learning difficulties are inherently due to difficulty with the subject and how much is directly attributable to dyslexia? Plenty of children who don't have dyslexia have trouble with maths, for example, and plenty more hate writing essays and dislike reading.

Those times when we just want to yell at our child to knuckle down or shape up, are the times when we force ourselves to reach deep inside and pull out a little more patience, love and understanding. Try to be patient with your child because life is certainly no easier from his perspective than it is from yours!

For his part, your child may be wrestling with the fears and problems that arise from living in a world where everyone except him seems to know what is going on. It is a world where peers in the child's classroom may be discussing the plot of a novel and he may feel like an outsider where everyone is speaking a foreign language. It can be terrifying for a child, and especially for an adolescent, to know that he is struggling with things that others find easy.

It is one thing to plan and theorise about arming your child with tools and tips to fight or accept dyslexia, and another altogether for your child to put these things into practice every day and try to make them work. He needs your help.

You can help your child achieve his maximum potential

When considering your dyslexic child's needs, it is important to pay attention to his whole being. There is much more to a child with dyslexia (or indeed any child) than how to learn academically. A successful learning environment for your child is one that nurtures every aspect of his physical, cognitive, social, emotional and spiritual well-being.

Taking a holistic approach will remove many of the obstacles in your child's path to a happy, productive and satisfying life. There are particular problems a child with dyslexia faces most children do not have to deal with. Many can be offset or avoided if you are able to recognise them, and plan counter-strategies for dealing with them, before they become overwhelming.

You have probably heard of Abraham Maslow and his hierarchy of needs.[46] Maslow developed his theory that we have a psychological priority for the order in which we fulfil our needs. To be well-adjusted and fulfilled human beings, we must meet the most basic physiological needs first. We cannot survive without food, water and shelter, for example. Our social needs are higher up the hierarchy. It is important for us to establish friendships and receive social acceptance, but if we are unable to provide ourselves with basic food and shelter, then our social needs take a back seat.

As parents, we provide a caring and nurturing environment for our children that is both physically and emotionally safe for them to grow up in. We naturally provide the basic needs in Level 1 that Maslow talks about, until they are able to provide those things for themselves, but we also provide much more. We cannot attain self-actualisation for them, but we can set them up with the infrastructure of a happy home, where they are accepted for who they are and provide them with the right education, so that they will be in a good position to achieve their true potential as they develop into adults.

I have adapted Maslow's 5 levels of human needs to meet the learning needs of children by creating the ideal environment that enables your child to develop and learn effectively, achieve his maximum potential, and grow into a well-balanced, happy and self-fulfilled adult:

Fröhlich's Road to Success
Children's Holistic Needs

Level 1 – *Children's Basic Needs: Body, mind and soul*
Health, nutrition, water, quality sleep, exercise, warm loving home, learning through play, unconditional love and stress-free

Level 2 – *Happy Home: Safety and acceptance*
Feeling protected, supported at school, supported at home, feeling understood and being yourself

Level 3 – *Loving Relationships: Belonging*
Identifying your talents, loving yourself, loving family and good friends, being part of a group or community and loving others

Level 4 – *Self-esteem: Self-respect*
Pride, achievement in and out of school, celebrating success, respect from others, encouragement and praise

Level 5 – *Your True Potential: Achieving happiness*
Freedom to explore and understand, using your talents, being creative, doing what you love and achieving inner peace

---

In my view, children require more basic needs at the first level than those of Maslow, to provide an ideal learning environment. My holistic approach, 'Road to Success', therefore considers the needs of a child with dyslexia across all five levels, especially at the very basic Level 1.

Fröhlich's Road To Success
Children's Holistic Needs

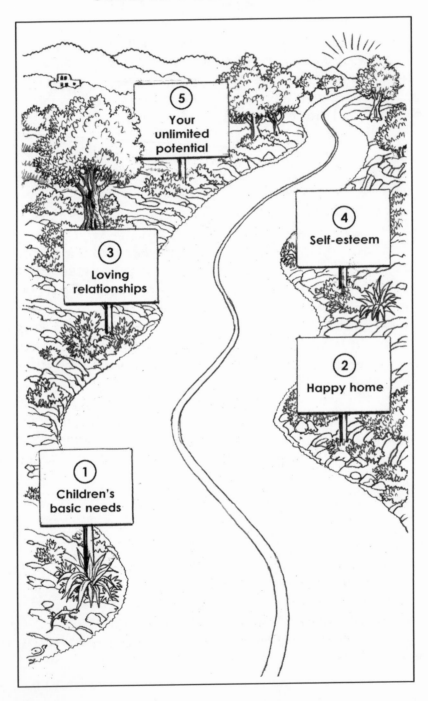

Level 1: Children's Basic Needs

Body, Mind and Soul:

- Health
- Nutrition
- Water
- Quality sleep
- Exercise
- Warm loving home
- Learning through play
- Unconditional love
- Stress-free

The basic level of needs is our physiological or biological one, such as food, water, sleep, exercise and good health, so that we can maintain a stable inner environment. When our basic needs are not satisfied, our inner energy is consumed by trying to rectify any imbalances and our survival instinct kicks in and goes into fight–flight mode. All other needs are irrelevant until we have a firm foundation and satisfy our most basic physiological needs.

While children do make progress at school, that progress can be limited by not addressing a basic need, and they may not be reaching their potential. Sometimes it is difficult to detect that our basic needs are not fully satisfied, but I focus on them in the following subsections.

As well as Maslow's identification of these basic needs, I believe all children need to do what young children do naturally and instinctively: play, laugh, run about, learn and feel loved. This is best done in a happy, stress-free environment. Laughter, play, exercise and learning are basic essential rights for all our children if they are to develop a sense of self and begin to flourish. Love is paramount at all levels.

Without these basic needs, children cannot learn effectively and the higher-level needs become more difficult to attain.

Level 1 – Health

Any medical needs your child has that produce discomfort, pain or suffering clearly need to be taken care of before he is in a position to learn effectively. Children with dyslexia are more susceptible to distraction than those without, and feeling unwell or having an illness is a serious distraction. Your child will not be firing on all cylinders.

In the chapter **What causes dyslexia?**, I focus on auditory and visual processing issues and retained primitive reflexes that seem to be prevalent in children with dyslexia. Start by establishing whether your child is experiencing any such barriers to learning, and take corrective action.

Under normal circumstances, your child will have his fair share of coughs and colds but, over the years, I have noticed that tummy aches and feeling 'unwell' seem to be quite prevalent in children with learning challenges. Always have this checked out by a doctor to rule out anything serious. In many cases, stomach aches and headaches can be due to anxiety, stress or low self-esteem and may present as symptoms of anxiety that should not be ignored and which are very real for your child. They are a cry for help. Once you have confirmed there is no medical reason for the tummy ache, try and get to the bottom of what is causing the stress, for example, friendship or family issues or low grades. In the section **Developing high self-esteem,** I offer many relaxation/therapies to help your child.

There are other physical considerations that can hold children back from being at their best:

- Feeling too cold
- Feeling too hot
- Feeling hungry
- Feeling exhausted from school
- Feeling irritated by clothing: zips, labels or fabrics
- Distraction from background noise
- Dislike of certain food tastes or textures
- Sensitivity to touch

Level 1 – Nutrition

While there is no magic pill to cure dyslexia, there is evidence that proper nutrition can help. Dyslexia is a biological condition that is often inherited and can be overcome, rather than eliminated, by carefully developed coping strategies that appeal to, and work in synergy with, a child's natural abilities and preferences. Nutrition plays an important part in being physically and mentally healthy and alert. Healthy food fuels children's brains and affects their life and learning power. We are what we eat.

> Good nutrition is important for all, especially for those younger than five years as these years are demanding for the developing child. They are the years in which children acquire many of the physical attributes and the social and psychological structures for life and learning.
>
> British Medical Association 2005

What is and is not acceptable nutritionally has shifted several times in recent years. We have seen recommendations come and go about diets rich in protein and low in carbohydrates, low-fat diets or vegetarianism. No matter what the recommended diet *du jour*, the evidence is clear that, in the modern age, with both parents working and limited time to stop and cook proper meals, convenience foods may dominate many people's diets.

A mounting body of evidence suggests that a deficiency in essential fats such as the important omega-3 and omega-6 fatty acids can contribute to brain dysfunction. A study of 97 children with dyslexia, performed by Dr Richardson and colleagues at Hammersmith Hospital in London[47], found that children with dyslexia and dyspraxia tended to be deficient in omega-3 and omega-6 fats. Several studies are also mentioned by Food for the Brain.[48]

Omega-3 fats are found in vegetable oils such as olive oil and soybean oil, egg yolks, and oily fish such as tuna and salmon. Omega-6 fats are also found in vegetable oils, green vegetables and nuts. The eyes require a high concentration of essential fats to perform efficiently the very rapid eye movements that occur when processing visual information. Research has found that 20% of the brain and 30% of the eye retina is comprised of such fats.

The body of evidence continues to grow that essential oils are important for us all. While we cannot argue yet that oil supplements will 'cure' dyslexia, dyspraxia or ADHD, research definitively suggests that omega-3 and omega-6 oils are a nutritious and vital ingredient in any diet and can be of great help to children or adults with learning disabilities that are a result of brain function.

If your child dislikes fish, eggs or other foods rich in omega-3 and -6, you can try supplements (from most supermarkets or health food stores), usually in the form of fish oils, but also in other vegetable oil combinations. They are not drugs or chemicals, but naturally occurring nutritious ingredients. Pumpkin seeds, flax seeds and flax seed oil, salmon, herring, tuna, kippers, eggs and olive oil are all rich in these healthy oils.

Besides healthy oils, make sure your child's diet is high in protein and brain-friendly complex carbohydrates (starch) – these are found in whole grains such as brown rice, pasta, potatoes, wholegrain cereals, wheat germ, oatmeal, beans, nuts and lentils. Minimise sugar and non-nutritious foods such as sweets (particularly if your child might be glucose intolerant or hyperactive).

Sugar, salt and preservatives are common ingredients found in almost all processed foods, and the bad effects of an over-abundance of these in our diets are well-understood. Sugar, preservatives and 'E' numbers mess up our digestive systems and are especially detrimental for children who have a tendency towards being hyperactive. Instead, look for easy ways to give unprocessed whole foods without preservatives or additives to all your family and all will benefit from the change.

For children who are susceptible to being hyperactive, having feelings of low self-esteem, depression or problems sleeping, a balanced nutritional diet is critical.

Serotonin plays an important role in relaxing the brain and low serotonin levels have been linked to lack of concentration, sleeplessness, depression, obesity and migraine. Our levels of serotonin are affected by natural light and by the foods we eat.

When our serotonin levels are low, we feel depressed; when they are high, we feel happier.

Our body doesn't get serotonin from foods but makes it from tryptophan, which is an essential amino acid that our body needs for normal growth in children and nitrogen balance in adults. Foods high in tryptophan include cheese, eggs, milk, nuts (walnuts), peanut butter, pumpkin seeds, sesame seeds, soy and tofu; bananas, pineapples, kiwis, tomatoes, spinach, avocados, asparagus; fish (cod, tuna, halibut), beef, chicken, turkey and pork. Our serotonin levels are vital to good mental and physical health.

Be on the lookout also for food allergies. These are exceptionally difficult to diagnose but can cause physical havoc to those of us who suffer from them. Food allergies are often at the root of conditions such as eczema. If you suspect a food allergy such as a wheat, dairy or gluten intolerance, try eliminating them from your child's diet one at a time, over a period of time, noting any physical or emotional changes, or see a food allergy specialist.

Level 1 – Water

Our body is more than 60% water and our brains comprise around 70% water. We all know the importance of drinking about two litres of water a day, but most of us fail to do so. Children physically need water to grow, as well as to improve mental agility. Many studies highlight the benefit of drinking water to improve cognitive performance in terms of memory, concentration and performance, in the classroom, in tests and on the sports field.

Although many children would rather drink squashes or fizzy drinks than water, do explain the benefits of drinking water to your child and encourage him to carry a bottle of water in his rucksack.

Level 1– Quality sleep

Quality sleep is important for effective learning, in particular for children with dyslexia, who need to concentrate hard. Many parents say that their child finds it difficult to get to sleep;

conversely, others say that their child is always tired and needs more sleep than most. Sleep is a basic Maslow need, and it's an obvious one. But *quality* sleep and the process of gently winding down before bedtime can sometimes be overlooked.

Children with learning difficulties become exhausted at school – they are putting in much more effort and concentration than children who do not find learning a problem. Many children find it difficult to wind down after a busy or stressful day because they are over stimulated or over exhausted. Some physical exercise or activity after school is good to reenergise or unwind from school, but some children do too many after-school activities, which wipes them out. They also need time to relax at home.

Early nights are vital. Many children say they are not tired when, in fact, they are overly wound up, and a lack of routine at bedtime means they don't sleep well at night. I recommend including a ritual in the bedtime routine to wind down and relax, such as having a warm bath, listening to an audio book, reading a book to your child, or having your child read to you, or playing calming background music.

Computer games, TV or electronic reading books over stimulate children's minds, and suppress melatonin, the sleep hormone, so I would make sure that children don't use any form of technology or electronic gadgets two hours before bedtime, so that they have a good night's sleep.

Level 1 – Exercise

One of the main benefits of exercise and physical activity generally is that it forces the body to increase its oxygen supply. Oxygen, like water, is essential to life. We know that an increase in oxygen is beneficial in almost any physical ailment. For example, it has been proven that an increase in oxygen can help a wound to heal faster. It is also widely accepted that providing more oxygen to the brain increases alertness and response times. The benefits of sport go way beyond the physical advantages of increasing the body's oxygen supply, and can have a positive impact on a child's emotional well-being, self-esteem and general competence in life.

Exercise is good for the brain

Perhaps the single biggest benefit of exercise and sport for dyslexic students is that it provides an outlet for letting off steam. Frustration is one of the things that dyslexic learners at school suffer from the most. Sport is a healthy and fun outlet for releasing stress.

Doing physical activity not only takes your mind off anything that is bothering you, but also releases feel-good endorphins that make you happy. Scientists are currently theorising that not only can exercise improve memory and release endorphins, but it can lead to the generation of new neurons.[49] Also, the generation of new neurons occurs in the brain's hippocampus, which means that they directly benefit learning and memory.

Exercise will also improve poor coordination skills, which are a common characteristic of children with dyslexia, dyspraxia and other learning difficulties. These skills are divided into two categories: gross and fine motor control.

Gross motor skills involve the coordinated effort of the large muscles of the body. Children with learning difficulties or other medical conditions may have poor or delayed gross motor skills, which affect their whole body (running, jumping, throwing, swimming), balance and motor planning.

Fine motor skills involve the ability to use the smaller muscles in the body for precise tasks that involve hand–eye coordination and gripping, such as writing, drawing, tracing and using scissors. If your child has any difficulties in these areas, I would recommend that you visit an occupational therapist or physiotherapist to assess his individual needs and advise you.

Level 1 – Home environment

Children have little control over their environment, internal or external, and rely on us to provide a loving and nurturing physical and emotional environment. Adults are more able to cope with sensitivities to heat/cold, noise, lighting, darkness, smells, vibes and the general atmosphere in the home than children are. Usually, children don't understand their sensitivities and are, therefore, unable to communicate that their environment is adversely affecting them. This negative impact can manifest itself through bad behaviour, lack of concentration, poor attention, stress, anger – some of which are a cry for help.

It's worth paying attention to the finer details of your child's general comfort, because the benefits of an ideal home environment that facilitate learning cannot be overestimated.

Level 1 – Learning through play

I would like to underline the importance of play for children *of any age*, including recreational and leisure activities as part of 'playtime' for older children, teenagers and adults. In fact, we all need time to 'chill out' and be away from the important things we have to take care of every day. Everyone needs time to rest their brain, and time out to pursue hobbies or frivolous activities, or simply to let their imaginations run away with them.

Many educators, scientists and advocates concerned with the welfare of children considered play so important that they formed the International Play Association (IPA), whose objective is to 'protect, preserve and promote the child's right to play as a fundamental human right'. The IPA refers to four important rights of children.[50]

> Every child has the right to rest and leisure, to engage in play and recreational activities appropriate to the age of the child.

There is a mounting consensus among psychologists and educators that all forms of play, and free play especially, are vital in helping children develop emotionally, academically, cognitively, socially and intellectually. Evidence suggests that both group play and individual play are fundamental to the all-round well-being of children, and both offer different benefits. Group play is more social, whereas individual play is more calming.[51]

Consequently, play is more than just fun for children - it is an essential part of how they learn. Children and teenagers use play to explore ideas and solve problems. They also use it to learn about relationships between things and relationships between people. They use it to develop their creative and physical skills and manual dexterity. Playing encourages social interaction and language development. It is as true for teenagers and adults as it is for young children (although adults sometimes forget how to play).

The rules for social interaction that children learn when playing together can set the stage for how they get along in the real world as they grow up. Playing also encourages children to learn skills they need to master for dealing with real life. For example, dressing and undressing a doll can help a small child learn to manipulate various fastenings; and colouring with crayons encourages children to fine-tune their fine motor skills.

Running and jumping, or kicking a ball around, provides valuable exercise, builds muscle, burns off energy and can lead to a genuine interest in athletic activities. Mastering physical activities such as riding a bike or swimming can build self-esteem and foster a feeling of growing independence and achievement. Captaining a football or hockey team can also foster leadership ability. Being a player on a football team, or a member of the chess team or the debating society is also a great way to experience positive peer pressure, enjoy the camaraderie of a team and experience safe exposure to healthy competition.

Play is an essential part of how we all learn

Play can also fulfil another important role in a child's life by providing an outlet for dreaming. Through play and imagination you can have things that life cannot provide. You can be a soldier, a princess or a policeman. You can rule the galaxy or navigate a starship through a dangerous black hole. You can be a racing car driver or plummet three thousand metres into a deep, dark ocean and meet scary creatures. All this leads to so much more than a healthy imagination. It can fuel motivation for things you want to do later in life and allows a child to develop a healthy emotional outlook.

As your child grows, the games can change to something more age appropriate – board games are always fun (and a great way to learn literacy and numeracy skills) and there are so many different types that you are sure to find something that appeals. Watching your child play (especially if you can observe unobtrusively) is a good way to find out what drives and motivates him and what kinds of things he enjoys doing. This can be especially useful for a child with dyslexia because it can provide clues about the kind of talent your child might unwittingly be demonstrating.

Knowing what your child is good at allows you to guide and encourage him when he feels fed up or frustrated with his dyslexia. Watching your child play, or playing with him, can help you draw out talents when there are tears, and convert the tears to laughter. Over the years, pursuing these talents can lead to increased self-esteem and true success.

Play impacts every aspect of a child's development. It is important to allow time for effective and unabashed playtime because it helps children discover who they are, what they like, and the ways of the world. It helps them develop social and problem-solving skills, and helps to expand and develop their knowledge of language, mathematics, science and the world around them. It inspires them to think creatively, develop their imagination and figure out where their talents lie. Play helps to develop leaders, organisers, followers, teachers, musicians and artists. It also brings much joy and happiness and a chance to try different roles and personalities on the way to becoming the best possible version of oneself.

As children get older, it may appear that they are spending too much time doing instant messaging with their friends, texting or talking on the phone – and that they are putting off doing their homework. But striking a balance between giving your teen 'chill out/play' time and keeping up with homework is a vital component in ensuring their emotional health.

Teenagers are still learning while playing (as we all are until the day we die). Playing for teens consists of much social interaction with peers, talking and debating, teasing each other, sports, and group activities such as outings to the cinema or shops, all of which help teens develop social skills and tune in to body language, moods and attitudes.

When children are playing, their minds are open to learning in a stress-free way. Parents and educators can leverage this fact when helping their dyslexic learners.

And don't forget about yourself. Mums and dads need to play too! As the busy parent of a demanding child, you too need plenty of time off, time out, quiet time, chill-out time and play time.

You may be interested to know about play therapy, which is an expressive therapy using a variety of toys, games and other media specifically chosen for their expressive qualities. It is a way of helping children aged 0 to 14 years express their feelings and deal with their emotional problems, using play as the main communication tool, such as drama, dance, movement, storytelling, visualisation, puppets, games, sand, clay, Plasticine™, painting and drawing, to name but a few.

Level 1 – Unconditional love

All children, especially those with learning difficulties, need unconditional love in the form of acceptance and recognition to reaffirm they are truly 'good enough' and, more important, that they meet or exceed our expectations. Children's mental well-being is as important as their physical well-being.

They are looking for our approval – unconditional love

As mentioned earlier, children who find learning difficult may suffer from headaches and stomach aches due to anxiety or anger. Children often don't meet their own expectations, and feel demoralised and sad about achieving low grades. They need continual praise for achieving small steps, and genuine acceptance for who they are. They are looking for our approval – unconditional love.

When children are loved unconditionally, they know that we are there for them no matter what. They know that we will do whatever we can to help them with their homework, revise for tests, read with them and play with them. Even when you discipline your child, they need to know it is out of love and that they are being protected from being hurt, or that you are teaching them moral values such as respect and helping them develop a sense of responsibility for themselves and others.

Unconditional love brings children a sense of security and provides them with the confidence to handle life's adversities. They instinctively know that all their basic needs are being met. Unconditional love makes children happy.

Level 2 Needs: Happy Home

Safety and Acceptance:

- Feeling protected
- Being supported at school
- Being supported at home
- Feeling understood
- Being yourself

Once we have satisfied the physiological needs, we seek protection and safety and a structure for law and order within our community. While not as essential as physiological needs, the need for a safe, stable environment is a fundamental learning need, both physically and emotionally.

As parents, we make it a priority to establish a good relationship with our children, with calm, understanding parenting methods and fond memories. A strong, positive relationship between parents and children is vital for children's self-confidence and for them to be successful. Conflict and tension in the home create fear, sadness, withdrawn behaviour, learning and school difficulties and can even cause depression within our children.

Children with dyslexia are sometimes at odds with the world of school: the learning environment can feel harsh and difficult. Your child needs help with learning coping strategies and managing his workload.

Getting help for school work will make your child feel that he is being supported and understood. It can be hard watching other children find learning so much easier. Your child may have spent long hours mastering a homework problem only to walk away with a 'D' or an 'E' grade. Then they find out that their classmate dashed off some homework twenty minutes before class started and got an easy 'A'.

Situations like this make it all the more important that your child comes home to an environment where he is not only comfortable and safe, but where he can be 'vulnerable', get cross, express his frustration, and vent his feelings about his learning difficulties or bad day at school. Try to set aside special one-to-one time together where you can chat and hear how his day has gone. You can discuss positive strategies to work through together to help him cope with any problems.

Siblings fight over the slightest thing at times; but if your younger child is reading at a higher level than your older child, for example, this can cause sibling rivalry and upset, along with some brutal comments. With a little understanding about how everyone has different strengths and weaknesses and pointing out the talents of your child with dyslexia, siblings can learn to be understanding and perhaps even helpful.

Routines make children feel safe by helping them learn to anticipate what will happen next, understand sequences of events and understand the relationship between cause and effect. A predictable routine allows children to feel safe, and to develop skills in handling their lives. As these life skills are strengthened, children can better tackle larger challenges.

In a happy environment, parents can deliver powerful messages about self-belief, belonging and love that will help children develop a great sense of self-discipline. Self-belief enables children to look at their perceived weaknesses and take steps to improve them.

Level 3 Needs: Loving Relationships

Belonging:

- Identifying your talents
- Loving yourself
- Loving family and good friends
- Part of a group or community
- Loving others

After we have assured our safety, we turn to ourselves and our relationships for love and acceptance. Family, social and working relationships are all important ingredients of belonging, as is the need to be a part of a community such as a church, school, club or sports team that extends beyond the immediate family and supports relationships with others.

Love really does make the world go round. The theme of love (understanding and acceptance) is a vital thread in raising a successful child throughout all the levels. Love is one of the most powerful energies on the planet.

Children's positive sense of self-worth also comes from loving themselves. It comes from understanding their strengths and accepting and managing their challenges. Helping children to identify their strengths and talents helps them understand themselves, value themselves and their important contribution to life and the community. I devote a whole chapter to identifying talents: **Road to your child's success – Part II**.

The feeling of belonging is vital to feeling loved and accepted. If children with dyslexia understand themselves, feel understood, are accepted for who they are, and are recognised as an important contributor to family life, they will feel safe and loved. When children feel safe, their hearts are more likely to be open and stress-free, and they will be more available to understand, learn and love themselves. Their sense of self becomes more in harmony with their inner world. As a result, children become more 'real', authentic and genuine in their relationships with themselves and others.

Level 4 Needs: Self-esteem

Self-respect:

- Pride
- Achievement in and out of school
- Celebrating success
- Respect from others
- Encouragement and praise

Further on our journey, we look for the respect of others, and self-respect to feed our self-esteem. This level includes the need for children to focus on their talents, look after their reputation, enjoy achievement and recognition and celebrate success.

High self-esteem helps children deal with problems, get on better with others and make the most of what life throws at them. Children rely on good feelings to help them grow in confidence and emotional stature.

Acceptance, respect and being valued nurtures feelings of belonging and self-respect. Feeling good about oneself and feeling satisfied foster a desire to achieve more, therefore, it is fundamental to give meaningful encouragement and praise regularly.

Recognition of any achievement in school provides a feel-good factor

For children with learning difficulties, who often feel under pressure and criticised for not doing well, regular praise and reinforcement of their ability to achieve is vital.

It is paramount to recognise academic and other success to promote a sense of self-respect and respect from others. Learning support at school and home is vital in ensuring high self-esteem. There is a positive correlation between children's self-esteem, their attainment at school and their behaviour.

I can't emphasise enough how recognition for any achievement at school in any subject or activity or for effort, progress, good leadership, team-playing or empathy towards peers is essential.

Furthermore, recognition of any achievement in school (as opposed to outside school, which is not necessarily acknowledged at school) provides a feel-good factor that fuels a desire to attend, enjoy school and learn. Being valued by one's peers at school increases one's motivation to achieve more.

Acknowledging and celebrating children's achievements enables children to recognise and value them too! Their level of self-esteem will have a vast influence on their success or failure.

Level 5 Needs: Your Unlimited Potential

Achieving happiness:

- Freedom to explore and understand
- Using your talents
- Being creative
- Doing what you love
- Achieving inner peace

Achieving our true potential is the need for personal growth, self-development, new challenges and freedom to explore and understand ourselves and our world: by doing what we love, being creative and using our talents.

We generally try to fulfil these needs after we have satisfied the needs at the lower levels; though, many adults with dyslexia have achieved greatness in spite of or because of not meeting basic needs. However, at some point there may come a time when a lack of basic needs, recognition, acceptance or self-love may affect how we handle self-actualisation.

Maslow maintained that our needs are so vital to us that they are practically instinctive. In other words, we don't necessarily make a conscious decision to ignore our personal development until after we have secured the means to provide a regular food supply for ourselves.

But this is what subconsciously happens. If we are unable to fulfil a need, we feel deprived and unsatisfied. If we are unable to fill one or more of our most basic needs, we cannot function properly.

The ultimate goal for our children is that they realise their full potential and achieve happiness. All children have massive, unlimited potential within. Enabling children to reach their true potential can bring pleasure and personal fulfilment, and contributes to better physical and mental well-being.

Fröhlich's Road to Success is an important piece of the puzzle in helping children with dyslexia become successful. If the road is built on strong foundations and each layer is successfully put in place, an environment where children feel encouraged and supported is more likely to generate an inner confidence that accomplishment is attainable and this will feed your child's determination to be successful and happy.

Learning at school can be very difficult for children with dyslexia. Those who will succeed are the ones who are well supported, feel good about themselves, are motivated, and never lose sight of their identity, abilities and talents. Helping our children identify, develop and channel their talents is a fundamental element on the road to their success.

Chapter 10
Road to your child's success – part II: identifying children's talents

During residency, I recognized that I had dyslexia. And then I realized I had this gift for imaging. Radiology is where I belonged. I live in a world of patterns and images and I see things that no one else sees. Anomalies jump out at me like a neon sign.

Beryle Benacerraf, M.D. physician[52]

Children with dyslexia have so many positive qualities, gifts and talents, such as the ability to think 'outside the box'. They use their creativity to solve a wide variety of problems. Their aptitude for lateral thinking and creative problem solving is relevant in almost any situation. There are successful people with dyslexia in all walks of life. When an individual with dyslexia is trained or experienced in something requiring a certain aptitude or skill, who knows what can result from the powerful combination of education and imagination? I believe that every child has a special talent.

Every child has a special talent

Wonderful dyslexic qualities

If your child has developed an idea that he is 'not as good' as some other children in his class, while that may be true (at the moment) for reading, spelling or writing, it may be untrue for maths, science, visionary thinking, art, music, sports or a host of other things. Reading and comprehension happen to be among the first things measured and assessed in children, because they are fundamental to learning. But finding reading or school work difficult can lower self-esteem from a very early age.

So, if your child is not feeling good about himself at school, it is important to help him build up his self-confidence and self-esteem by discovering together what his wonderful qualities are: what he is good at and has a passion for. Knowing he is really good at something is a feel-good factor that gives a greater sense of self-belief, courage and determination to persevere with more challenging areas.

People with dyslexia are often good at visualisation, which is why they often prefer pictures and images to words and text. They can often visualise well in three dimensions and go on to become great architects or designers. They also make good artists, painters and sculptors and are imaginative writers. Even though your child may not immediately exhibit strong writing skills, do not rule out the possibility of a career that requires the ability to write well, using his great imagination. Countless authors have dyslexia – it is imagination that counts. Do open up horizons and possibilities and see where it leads.

People with dyslexia can also be great at mechanical engineering or design projects that are very hands-on. They are often good at sports, drama, dance, singing or music. Many famous actors, scientists and entrepreneurs have dyslexia. You may well already have a good feel for what your child is good at. If not, I encourage you to observe your child at a play or at work with new eyes, looking for signs of hidden or undiscovered talent. Then you can help him find outlets to use and develop these talents.

I recently read a children's book called *The Wind Singer*[53] so I could help children with their English essays. One part of the story that struck me was about residents of a city who are divided into groups according to how well they perform in 'The High Examination'. Hanno, a loving father who is rebelling against taking the exam, has been locked up and discovers that all the inmates have failed 'the test', but each one is a genius at something. One of them loves weather and can name all types of cloud formations. Another, a tailor, knows how to identify any kind of fabric by touch, and another, a janitor, seems to have no talent at all, but loves dipping biscuits in tea at lunchtime. He turns out to be a brilliant baker who can make a biscuit with just the right texture to be dipped into tea.

The story emphasises my point that we can become interested and brilliant in any subject area. There is a wide career field in almost any topic. In music, for example, besides working live on stage, in front of the camera or behind the camera, there are multiple opportunities for working in a sound-recording studio, television studios, record company, radio station or theatre.

If your child is good at music, discuss possible careers that can leverage musical skills. If your child demonstrates talent in non-core subjects such as geography or history, there is a multitude of professions that depend on those subjects. With a little research, you can help him uncover a splendid array of different careers to leverage just about any set of skills.

So encourage your child to use all that natural creativity that people with dyslexia possess to imagine all the possibilities and pursue the talents that he loves and which are naturally easy for him. Most important, provide your child with chances to discover what he is good at, and help him with positive encouragement when he shows a natural tendency for something – whatever it is. We are all happiest when we are doing what we like and what we have natural talent for, so let your child have fun exploring his own abilities and take delight in what comes naturally.

Indicators of children with high learning potential, and gifted and talented children

In school, being gifted usually refers to academic ability; being talented generally refers to exceptional performance in a non-academic subject. Not everybody is 'gifted' in the academic sense, or talented with an 'exceptional performance', but I firmly believe that **everyone** is talented in something – some to a greater extent than others.

**Attitude is the difference between
an opportunity and a problem**

One indicator of talent is an early enthusiastic interest in an area that does not fade as your child grows older. This is best described as passion for something such as sport, art, drama or dance, or the desire to learn a musical instrument. A child who is talented at something may strive to practise it all the time. You may never have to tell children who have a natural gift to practise or to hone their skills – they are probably already doing so under their own steam.

Accompanying this passion is a certain attitude. Failure or difficulty, rather than defeating them, seems to drive them forward. This attitude may ripple over to other areas where they are not so gifted. On the other hand, a student gifted at maths can have a good attitude in that subject, yet need cajoling to write an English essay.

Perhaps your child is not an 'A' student, but regularly gets an 'A' in one or more favourite subjects. This, too, can be an indicator of giftedness. A child who excels at track and field, rather than maths or English, may not receive the same sort of attention as a child gifted at academic subjects. That is where you can recognise your child's talent, encourage him to pursue it and reassure him that, despite having trouble with reading, he is talented in other areas.

Hobbies also are great indicators of giftedness or talents. If we find a way to turn our hobbies into our careers, we tend to be fulfilled and happy individuals.

Some children are natural leaders and rally their friends to form clubs. Recognise an entrepreneurial spirit in a child who is always looking for ways to make money, whether by selling his old games on eBay, or knocking on neighbours' doors and asking to mow their lawn or wash the car. Some children are gifted storytellers and make comic books, write stories or enchant their friends with tales in which imagination plays a significant role. Others love to draw everything new they encounter. Perhaps your child cannot put down a ball, or plays a musical instrument for hours?

A curious child who is driven to find answers to questions may turn out to be a great researcher or explorer. A child who collects insects in the garden or seeks out plants and flowers and presses or catalogues them is indicating curiosity.

These tell-tale signs are all areas of higher learning potential that you can nurture and encourage. Helping your child to recognise and understand where his talents lie is one of the best things you can do to help him on his way to a fulfilling life. It helps him understand himself and gives him something to hold on to when he has difficulty with spelling or grammar or finds himself unable to read out loud in class.

Potential Plus UK is a fantastic organisation that supports the social, emotional and learning needs of children of all ages and backgrounds with high learning potential (previously known as the National Association of Gifted Children – NAGC) **www.potentialplusuk.org.uk**. Nowadays, the term High Learning Potential (HLP) is preferred to terms such as 'gifted', 'gifted and talented' or 'more able/very able' learners.

Take a look at the table of indicators of children with high learning potential. Do you recognise any of these indicators in your child?

Indicators of Children with High Learning Potential[54]
• Is always asking questions
• Is extremely curious
• Gets involved physically and mentally
• Has unusual or silly ideas
• Is the class joker
• Fiddles with things and messes about
• Plays around in class, yet tests well
• Questions the answers
• Is often beyond the ability of any age peer group
• Shows strong feelings and opinions
• Already knows the answer, but often doesn't know how
• Needs 1–2 repetitions to master a concept
• Constructs abstract theories

- Prefers the company of adults or older children
- Draws inferences from things that don't seem connected
- Initiates projects
- Is intense
- Has a strong sense of justice and right and wrong
- Creates a new design
- Enjoys learning new things (not going over the same things!)
- Applies/manipulates information
- Is an inventor
- Is good at guessing
- Thrives on complexity
- Is keenly observant
- Is highly self-critical

Identifying and channelling the talents of children with dyslexia

Howard Gardner developed the theory of Multiple Intelligences[55] because he believed we are intelligent in many different ways. (I talk about this in more detail in the **Learning Preferences and Multiple Intelligences** chapter.) It is also important to apply Gardner's theories in understanding where children's talents lie. Some of us are more proficient at some of the intelligences and some are more proficient at others.

It is rare to find individuals who do not exhibit a tendency to be good in *any* of the areas of intelligence. Many people (both with and without dyslexia) exhibit proficiency in more than one area. We can summarise the intelligences as:

- verbal-linguistic
- logical-mathematical
- musical-rhythmic

- visual-spatial
- kinaesthetic
- interpersonal (being good with other people)
- intrapersonal (understanding yourself, or having a high quotient of emotional intelligence)
- naturalist (good at biology, science, nature)
- existential (interested in philosophical issues of life)

The table Identifying Your Child's Talents will help you recognise which talents and strong interests your child has and you may discover a pattern or tendency towards certain skills. The contents are not exhaustive, but provide you with a sample to add to. We are often best at the things we love, and most satisfied in our work when we are doing things we enjoy that leave us feeling satisfied.

Talk to your child about dyslexia. Make sure he understands it is not a disease and that many people have dyslexia; while it may present some challenges, it may also open many doors. Help your child appreciate the talents he has and teach him how to become a well-rounded individual by focusing on strengths while continuing to persevere at developing weaker areas.

Even though many children with dyslexia have a dislike of books and reading, you can still provide a steady and varied supply of books on interesting subjects that have plenty of pictures, or are interactive. Even older children still enjoy books with pictures. For example, for a child interested in football, a colourful annual or mini encyclopaedia with photographs of his favourite players, or famous players, might captivate his attention and encourage him to read more.

Similarly, activities that encourage building, creation and interaction, such as jewellery kits, train sets, painting by numbers and craft sets do not have to be reserved for smaller children. Visit a hobby shop and purchase adult versions to encourage teenagers to pursue the things they loved to do as youngsters.

If your young child demonstrates an interest in music, explore musical toys before investing in the more expensive real versions. If your child is interested, try music lessons to see how they go. If you have to tell your child to practise, or there is not much progress after several months, do not force the issue; becoming a virtuoso may not be for him.

Identifying Your Child's Talents and Gifts		
Musical instrument	Singing	Dance
Drama	Cooking	Sewing
Woodwork	Team sport	Individual sport
Horse riding	Athletics	Swimming
Martial arts	Gymnastics	Cycling
Graphics	Technology	Design
Painting	Drawing	Crafts
Magic	Fashion	Photography
Board games	Gardening	Chess
Nature	Animals	3-D construction
Humour	Mechanics	Driving
Emotional awareness	Social skills	Ideas and imagination
Intuition	Leadership	Problem solving
Business	Maths	Science
Reading	Writing	Speaking
History	Geography	Religious studies
Foreign languages	Debating	General knowledge

If your child is still young (well, any age in fact and even adults), reading to him can help to stimulate ideas and discussions as well as expose him to a variety of subjects, educational concepts and stories that are fun and inspirational. Reading to children with dyslexia is especially beneficial because they miss out by not reading (or not wanting to read) as much as other kids. Reading, or listening to someone read, exposes them to vocabulary and grammar and opens up their world to things they may never experience in everyday life. For example, a child who does not read or pay attention in school may not know the animals of Africa, the countries of the world or the planets in the solar system. Not only does this make his world smaller, but it may make him feel vulnerable in school when he does not know simple things that other children take for granted.

Reading, or being read to, also gives children ideas. It gives them space to let their imaginations soar and build dreams. It can also be a great way to unwind after a long night of doing homework or struggling at school with a new subject or a spelling test. Listening to someone else read a story is relaxing and calming, and allows them to experience the joy of a story without the struggle of reading it themselves. I still love being read to.

Social play and imagination can be a great strength. Playing with other children, by oneself or with an imaginary friend should never be considered a waste of time; rather, it is an important aspect of child and teenage development and nurtures creativity.

Imagination can be a great strength

Listening to music or watching documentaries is also a way of stimulating the imagination. Many famous movie producers and actors made up their minds to pursue their professions after being inspired by a favourite film or documentary. I am not suggesting that you let your child sit in front of a TV for hours, but don't ban good programmes completely – what if your child is destined to become the next Walt Disney or David Attenborough?

Many children with dyslexia prefer to be up and moving or doing, rather than sitting back and listening or watching, so the problem of watching too much TV may not even surface. While your child is young enough (and it's not 'uncool') to enjoy going on nature walks with you, exploring parks and trails, going to the zoo or the aquarium, and visiting museums, encourage this. It allows you to interact with one another, be around people, explore nature and learn about the past and, most of all, provides a variety of scenarios for your child to discover what kinds of things motivate him and stimulate his imagination. It gives you a wider variety of settings in which to observe your child and see what makes him tick. You also get to enjoy each other's company in a relaxed way.

Parents of children with dyslexia often report that their children do not like school and even getting them to go to school can be challenging. But it does not necessarily follow that every child with dyslexia will not like school, particularly if they focus on what they are good at.

I have a friend whose son has dyscalculia. He finds maths and science quite challenging, yet excels at French and music, and plays the cello in the school orchestra. He loves school, not just because he is good at playing the cello, but because he is highly sociable and enjoys the interaction with his peers. He considers school a social place and gets enjoyment from having good friends. This child is gifted socially. He is a good listener, easy to talk to and interested in a wide variety of conversational topics, and interacts well with adults. Despite this social giftedness and his intelligence, he continues to get Ds in maths and science and frequently forgets to hand in his homework.

By the same token, it does not follow that a child who does not enjoy school is not talented and has no hope for the future. It means that, for whatever reason, your child is not enjoying school. Try to find out the exact reason for this. Just as my friend's son enjoyed school for social reasons, a child may not enjoy school for a reason that is completely unrelated to academic issues.

Giftedness refers to the inherent natural talents that children or adults are born with. However, even if a natural talent has not yet emerged, it can be awakened, nurtured and enhanced with the right kind of encouragement at school and at home. Reportedly, children who have a computer at home regularly do better in school than children who do not. Children whose parents religiously attend every dance recital or football game regularly do better at sports than children whose parents do not take an interest in extra-curricular activities.

Children do best when they feel encouragement rather than pressure

As parents, we find it difficult to assess whether we are achieving the result of positive encouragement or putting our children under pressure. The only way to know for sure is to ask your child. Don't be afraid of asking him if he feels under pressure. Some children are more aware than others of the pressures and stresses they face, and some are more able to articulate it than others. Children do best when they feel encouragement rather than pressure.

If you have an open communication with your child and can discuss things freely, he will be able to tell you whether you are unwittingly putting pressure on him. The point is to help him build confidence in his strengths in order to develop his potential – whatever that might be – and enable him to persevere in his weaker areas so that he can improve, not necessarily excel, by doing the best he can without undue difficulty.

Parental influence is of critical importance for children. Even though peer pressure can be phenomenally influential, do not underestimate your power as a parent to be a defining influence on your child's belief in himself. Children with dyslexia often quote their parents' unfailing belief in them as the main reason why they were able to overcome their challenges in spite of being told by some teachers that they would never amount to anything. Your belief in them will make them feel terrific. I know for a fact that my children feel this way.

If children with dyslexia exhibit giftedness in an academic subject that features prominently in the school curriculum, it can be hard for parents to decide whether to encourage them to pursue it at a higher level. What if they fail? What if the reading and writing demands are more than they can handle? Don't be afraid of encouraging your child to pursue some subjects to higher levels if the opportunity arises. Look on the positive side. A child who feels constantly defeated by, say, reading, can feel the universe has no bounds if he also excels at science or art, and increased self-esteem is the direct result if he can attain a higher level of achievement in a subject he enjoys.

Preventing underachievement in high potential learners

We need to be aware of our children's gifts and talents, so that they perform to their potential and do not underachieve. High potential learners who are not stretched in the classroom will become bored, demotivated and not reach their potential.

Children who are not stretched may become fed up, angry or depressed and find it difficult to complete school assignments. They may begin to misbehave and develop social or emotional problems. They may even refuse to attend school and drop out at the earliest opportunity. High potential children need to be stretched or they will suffer from low self-esteem.

Reasons Why High Learning Potential Children Can Sometimes Underachieve

- Inability to manage time
- Disorganised and frequently losing things
- Lack of intrinsic motivation to succeed
- Problems with friendships – either lack of friends or communication issues
- Bullying
- Disruptive, confrontational or disrespectful in class
- Difficulty concentrating either due to boredom or as yet undiagnosed Special Educational Need
- Poor handwriting and overall poor presentation of work
- Perfectionist personality type – resulting in purposely resisting work that is deemed more challenging as the fear of failure outweighs the glory of success

---

If you look at the tables 'Reasons why High Learning Potential Children can sometimes underachieve' and 'Characteristics of Underachieving High Potential Learners' and compare these characteristics to those of children with learning difficulties such as dyslexia or ADHD, you may think there are some similarities. And you would be right.

So what does that tell us? To me, it suggests that sometimes high learning potential children display qualities or traits we mistake for bad behaviour or inability to do the work when, in fact, they are not being challenged in the right way or may have a learning difficulty. This is another reason to have your child assessed, in order to get to the bottom of what is causing his misbehaviour or underachievement.

Characteristics of Underachieving High Potential Learners[56]

- Poor test performance
- Achievement at or below expectations in one of or all the basic skill areas
- Daily work frequently incomplete or poorly done
- Superior comprehension and retention of concepts when interested
- Vast gap between level of oral and written work
- Exceptionally large repertoire of factual knowledge
- Vitality of imagination: creative
- Persistent dissatisfaction with work accomplished, even in art
- Avoidance of trying new activities, to prevent imperfect performance; evidence of perfectionism, self-criticism
- Shows initiative in pursuing self-selected projects at home
- A wide range of interests and possible special expertise in an area of investigation and research
- Evidence of low self-esteem with tendencies to withdraw or be aggressive in the classroom
- Does not function comfortably or constructively in a group of any size
- Shows acute sensitivity and perceptions related to self, others and life in general

- Tends to set unrealistic self-expectations: goals too high or too low

- Dislikes practice work or drill for memorisation and mastery

- Easily distracted; unable to focus attention and concentrate efforts on tasks

- Has an indifferent or negative attitude towards school

- Resists teacher efforts to motivate or discipline behaviour in class

- Has difficulty in peer relationships: maintains few friendships

Affirming children's talents

It is important to acknowledge children's talents and encourage them in and out of school without pushing or exhausting them. It is equally important to affirm children for who they are even if they have not yet discovered their talent. Some of us are late bloomers and our special talents develop later in life. Children need to feel that they are loved unconditionally and that our love is not connected to their accomplishments. Then, when we take pride in their accomplishments, it comes with true meaning and freedom from pressure to live up to parental expectations. Likewise, if we are trying to guide or help children improve their natural talents, it will be easier if they already feel supported, loved and accepted for who they are at the core.

PART FOUR
Our Children's Education

Chapter 11
Learning preferences and multiple intelligences

Tell me and I forget, show me and I
remember, involve me and I understand.

Ancient Chinese proverb

Much work has been done by educators and psychologists in the last 100 years or so regarding the way children learn. From this research, two important points have become widely accepted:

- There are several stages that children go through as they grow, and they learn differently at different stages, so age-appropriate instruction is important in educating children.

- There are several ways that people learn, called the learning modalities (styles or preferences), that is, the different ways in which we learn. We do not all use the same style of learning in equal proportions. Teaching should therefore use a variety of methods, including visual, auditory and kinaesthetic, in order to reach every child.

Learning stages

Let's discuss the above two concepts in a little more depth. Jean Piaget was one of the leading developmental psychologists of the twentieth century. His work in cognitive development has been widely acclaimed and still forms the basis of our understanding today of how children's minds develop. Further in this chapter, I talk about learning preferences and how you can find the best learning style for your child who has dyslexia – just like all children, not all such children are the same, and trying a variety of learning styles will help you understand how your child learns best.

In order to develop strategies to help your child, it is useful to understand a little about the cognitive stages that children go through. These stages, while not hard and fast rules, are generally applicable to all children in a certain age group. Children's physical bodies and brains are still forming, as are their emotional intelligence, motor skills and their awareness of the world around them. Just as a small baby has to learn how to crawl before it can walk, so a baby's brain must learn to think in simple concepts before it can master complex, abstract ideas. In fact, the stage for abstract thinking is really an adult one, and does not appear in many children until the last years of secondary or high school.

There are four stages in Piaget's theory:

- The sensorimotor stage, which lasts from birth until about age 2;
- The preoccupational stage, which lasts from 2 to about 7;
- The concrete operational stage, which lasts from 6 or 7 until about 11;
- The formal operations stage, which develops around 11 and lasts into adulthood.

It is helpful to understand these stages because children learn differently in each one. Even if you are applying specific learning techniques for children with dyslexia, you need to be mindful of what a child of a certain age is capable of mastering cognitively, with or without dyslexia. I outline each stage briefly below.

1. Sensorimotor stage

From birth to age two, a child does not have control over its physical being, so this stage is largely concerned with gaining control of its movements and relating those movements to the world. Babies tend to put everything in their mouth in order to experience it yet, once an object is out of sight, young babies quickly forget about it. A baby also experiments with the idea that letting go of an object causes it to fall to the ground. Babies love to drop things! This is part of their learning experience.

2. Preoperational stage

Two- to seven-year-olds are learning to think symbolically. A three-year-old, for example, may remember a toy even after you have removed it from sight. At this stage, children are egocentric. They are not in tune with the fact that others have different feelings or different ideas from them. Social play is very important at this age as children begin to learn that other children have different opinions and different personalities.

Children of this age cannot process concepts logically as adults can. For example, a child may believe that it is cold in winter because it snows, rather than that it snows because it is cold in winter. At this age, showing children how something works is much better than telling them facts. For example, play with a glass of water and pour it into containers of different sizes and shapes to show them how a wide, shallow glass can hold as much water as a tall, thin one.

3. Concrete operational stage

Parents often realise their child has learning difficulties at the onset of this stage, which starts at around age 7 and lasts through primary school to 11 years. Children at this age begin to think in more logical terms and start to develop an understanding of how things work in reality.

In her book *Educational Psychology: Developing Learners* (2007), Jeanne Ellis Ormrod discusses how children process information differently. Children are presented with ten wooden beads, eight of which are brown and two of which are white. If you ask a four-year-old if there are more wooden beads than brown beads, he is likely to answer that there are more brown beads. A child of this age cannot comprehend that the white beads are also wooden beads. To a four-year-old, they are simply white. A ten-year-old, on the other hand, is likely to answer the question correctly; at this age, a child is capable of understanding that a bead can be both white and wooden. By then, children have also developed an understanding that it is possible to hurt people's feelings and that others think differently from them, but truly abstract thought still eludes them.

4. Formal operational stage

The ability to think logically or abstractly and the application of deductive reasoning begin to appear at 11–16 years onwards. There are people who never completely master this stage of development while others reach it early, depending on factors such as educational environment and inherent intelligence.

As we mature, we tend to concoct 'schemes' for organising our world. As we have new experiences, we fit them into our schemes. When the schemes no longer accommodate our experience, we develop more complex ones. By unconscious reference to our schemes of how the world works, we are able to apply deductive reasoning to problems and hypothesise about theories and solutions.

Learning in the classroom

Most secondary or high school children are in the early stages of formal operational development.

This stage of school education includes huge amounts of auditory (verbal) instruction, supplemented with handouts, textbooks and written material. Consequently, secondary school can be a challenging environment for young people with dyslexia, who often learn better from other teaching methods such as visual and kinaesthetic.

This is why these children often shine at science, art, drama, music, design and technology, sports and other physical activities, because their natural learning skills are more geared towards kinaesthetic than auditory learning. But please note there are many children with dyslexia who also shine in English, maths, history, geography, languages and other academic subjects.

Children with dyslexia learn best when teaching is personalised and targets more than one learning style

Teachers, therefore, can use a variety of teaching techniques in every subject to accommodate all the different learning styles. If you have a choice of where to send your child to school, it is worth finding out the teaching approaches and philosophies used by each school in your local area, as this can have a significant impact on your child's academic progress. There are guidelines about selecting schools in the chapter **Choosing the Right School**.

Laughter

Laughter benefits our mind, body and soul. Whoever said that 'laughter is the best medicine' had the right idea but was only scratching the surface regarding its benefits. There are both physiological and psychological benefits to a good belly laugh. Humour can break the ice, make any chore more fun, and make it easier to get along with people. Hearing other people laugh together instantly grabs our attention, and makes us hungry to hear what they find so funny.

Laughter benefits our mind, body and soul

Laughter makes us feel happy. When we laugh, our hearts literally open up, and it is really hard to feel stressed, frustrated or angry when we laugh. Some people say laughter cleanses our bodies and helps us learn by relaxing us and relieving stress. When a subject is presented with humour, it increases our interest as well as' our rapport with classmates and teachers. At the same time, we have improved memory retention (who wouldn't want to remember something that makes them laugh?) and, therefore, improved learning ability.

Laughter helps create a safe environment in which to learn

Ensuring that kids have plenty to laugh at during their day, or during the middle of a particularly difficult homework assignment, can go a long way to restoring them physically and mentally to a position where they are able to begin learning again. Laughter helps create a safe environment in which to learn.

The Power of Laughter

- Enhances your creative abilities and stimulates your problem-solving ability. Thinking up funny, outrageous, exaggerated or ridiculous things stretches your imagination, and a strong imagination is a great foundation for brainstorming and out-of-the-box thinking. Scientists have shown, using MRI scanning, this kind of thinking can actually stretch connections in the brain, link parts of the brain that would otherwise not be linked and enhance creative thinking.

- Helps defuse an embarrassing or 'heavy' situation, making it easier for people to deal with (so long as the subject of the laughter is in good taste and on a neutral subject).

- Helps strangers to bond and damaged relationships to heal.

- Helps to overcome feelings of shyness because it breaks the ice.

- Helps win people over – think about how people making a speech or delivering a lecture often start with a joke.

- Improves healing ability. Numerous studies corroborate evidence that laughing more often can help people heal physically.

- Improves memory retention because it becomes memorable.

- Improves your attention span because it grabs your attention – we all want to laugh.

- Increases learning ability because we want to participate.

- Increases self-confidence. A happy person is a confident person. When you laugh you feel happy.

- Reduces boredom when learning new things.
- Reduces stress and anxiety. The physical act of laughing causes the body to release endorphins, which gives us a feel-good factor. Laughing makes our muscles relax, and stress, which is primarily stored in the muscles, reduces as well.
- Strengthens your immune system by decreasing stress hormones and increasing immune cells and infection-fighting antibodies.

Humour in the classroom

Just as important in my mind as the physical implications of laughter is the fact that students relate much more readily to a teacher who uses laughter in the classroom and, when a child likes a teacher, he is more likely to learn from him or her.

When humour is used in the classroom, children are not just more likely to remember things but they also have more fun. Who doesn't want that for their children? Roars of laughter can be heard coming from my classroom, as I use humour to engage children and relieve their burden of stress about having to have extra support lessons. It makes them feel good about themselves.

Learning preferences (visual, auditory, read/write and kinaesthetic)

Modern psychologists have done a lot of work in this area and their research is helping us develop advanced teaching strategies for many so-called learning-challenged students. There are many ways to approach teaching and learning and if one way is not working well for your child, there is probably another way that will work better.

The modern rise of technology and the Internet has revolutionised the way we learn. Apart from everything else the computer provides, it puts several different approaches in easy reach of teachers and parents, and allows teachers to introduce, through the use of different computer programmes, several ways of teaching students who learn interactively.

A popular theory for learning approaches is the **V**isual, **A**uditory, **R**ead/Write, **K**inaesthetic (VARK) model introduced by Neil Fleming.[57] In the VARK model, one or two learning preferences are dominant in every individual and learning is most effective if you use the style each person prefers.

Visual, Auditory, Read/Write, Kinaesthetic (VARK) Learning Preferences	
Learning Preference	**Description**
Visual	Seeing
Aural/auditory	Listening and speaking
Read/write	Reading and writing
Kinaesthetic	Touching and doing

For example:

- Visual learners do well with aids such as diagrams, charts, patterns, graphs, videos and movies. You can identify this type of learner as being able to recall images and having a preference for pictures in books.

- Auditory learners like to listen to the teacher talk, or listen to books or lectures and discussion groups. This type of learner sometimes likes to move his lips when reading, or to read out loud.

- Read/write learners enjoy information displayed as words. This type of learner generally enjoys reading, and writing stories, essays and reports.

- Kinaesthetic learners prefer demonstrations, experiments or to experience and practise tasks. You can recognise this type of learner as enjoying personal experiences and creating things.

As many children with dyslexia seem to respond well to visual aids, if you send a child on an errand to a supermarket, he might do better with a picture of the product cut from a magazine, alongside the written word, than if you simply tell him the name of the product and expect him to remember and find it. Without a list or a picture, a child with dyslexia may forget what to buy, just as in this favourite old poem:

Going on an Errand[58]

A pound of tea at one and three
And a pot of raspberry jam
Two new laid eggs a dozen pegs
And a pound of rashers of ham.

I'll say it over all the way
And then I'm sure not to forget
For if I chance to bring things wrong
My Mother gets in such a sweat.

A pound of tea at one and three
And a pot of raspberry jam
Two new laid eggs a dozen pegs
And a pound of rashers of ham.

There in the hay the children play
They're having such fine fun
I'll go there too that's what I'll do
As soon as my errands are done

A pound of tea at one and three
A pot of er new laid jam
Two raspberry eggs with a dozen pegs
And a pound of rashers of ham.

There's Teddy White flying his kite
He thinks himself grand I declare
I'd like to make it fly up sky high
Ever so much higher than the old church spire

And then – but there

A pound of three at one and tea
A pot of new laid jam
Two dozen eggs, some raspberry pegs
And a pound of rashers of ham.

Now here's the shop outside I'll stop
And run my orders through again

I haven't forgot – it's better not
It shows I'm pretty quick that's plain.

A pound of tea at one and three
A dozen of raspberry ham
A pot of eggs with a dozen pegs
And a rasher of new laid jam.

Which learning preferences does your child favour?

People with dyslexia are least likely to prefer the read/write styles for obvious reasons. This style is favoured by many academics. Just because your child does not do well with this style of learning does not mean that he is not inherently intelligent. On the contrary, many people with dyslexia are exceptionally intelligent, but the emphasis on academic learning in school masks this fact because many schools, especially senior schools, tend to overuse the auditory learning style. That said, with the influx of interactive whiteboard presentations and 'live' environments, children have access to more visual, interactive information, provided it is presented in the correct fashion.

The learning preference of many dyslexic learners is kinaesthetic. With some imagination and creativity, you can think up ways to teach subjects in kinaesthetic ways that were traditionally regarded as academic. Think of physics and chemistry, for example: there is plenty of hands-on and experimentation in those subjects. The concept can easily be extended to other subjects. For example, imagine you are an English teacher and your challenge is to teach Shakespeare to a class that includes children with dyslexia. Would you choose to assign each child a character and have him or her read the play out loud in class? Or would you assign the children parts in a play and let them act out the important scenes? Allowing them to move the classroom furniture around to create different scenes, designing costumes or scenery will get them even more involved. Just imagine all the wonderful kinaesthetic ways we can teach history, geography or languages! It's much more fun for everyone, including the teacher.

The learning preference of many dyslexic learners is kinaesthetic

Kinaesthetic learners like to move around and take breaks. If they are compelled to sit still for long periods, they are likely to lose concentration. This can be especially true with dyslexic or ADHD learners. Kinaesthetic learners can be recognised by the fact that they are likely to sit and doodle, fidget and fiddle with things while they are listening. They will respond well to colourful charts and diagrams, coloured markers on a white board, interactive learning and demonstrations that include seeing, touch, taste, smell and movement. If you can work some music and rhythm into the lesson, that's better still. This is worth keeping in mind when you are working at home with your child.

Educators might favour the use of one learning style for one subject and another learning style for another subject. So drama class might be an interactive, kinaesthetic session, whereas maths might traditionally be more of a linguistic/logical intelligence approach (reading/writing/lecturing/ listening). The good news is that there is, generally, progress being made with respect to lesson plans that make better use of different learning styles in the classroom, especially kinaesthetic. The progress might possibly be too slow for your child, but it is good to know that there is a trend in the right direction.

Auditory sequential vs visual-spatial learners

Visual-spatial deals with spatial judgment and the ability to visualise with the 'mind's eye', i.e. experiencing visual mental imagery. Many people with dyslexia report that they are easily able to think and visualise in 3-D and are considered visual-spatial learners.

Two types of learners: auditory-sequential learners and visual-spatial learners

Dr Linda Kreger Silverman, in a report entitled Identifying Visual-Spatial and Auditory-Sequential Learners: A Validation Study[59], validates the point that there are primarily two types of learner: auditory-sequential, and visual-spatial learners. It may be fair to say that people without dyslexia often fall into the first category and many with dyslexia fall into the second. Auditory-sequential learners prefer to listen and can excel in phonemic awareness. They are often great communicators because they have good verbal fluency. For visual-spatial learners, learning comes most easily through images and pictures that represent a whole concept in a holistic fashion rather than processing small chunks of verbally communicated information.

Multiple intelligences

An important researcher in this area is Dr Howard Gardner, who introduced his theory of Multiple Intelligences in 1983. He originally listed seven, then eight, intelligences in the book and later added another one, so we talk about Gardner's nine intelligences. There is a table below.

Children with dyslexia often have trouble with linguistic intelligence, which includes speaking, listening, reading, writing and spelling. There is evidence to support the fact that the brain's processes in this area simply work differently in these children. The point to take away here is that if your child does not favour linguistic intelligence, there are *eight other intelligences you can appeal to in a child with dyslexia* (or any child) to enhance learning, and to which your child will probably respond better. Just because your child does not currently enjoy linguistic intelligence, does not mean he will not in the future. There are many successful authors who found reading, spelling, writing or speaking difficult when they were at school, who most certainly favour that intelligence now.

The trick is to figure out which learning preferences your child favours and then play into them

Taking multiple intelligences and learning preferences into consideration in the classroom is absolutely essential for children with learning challenges. As a specialist teacher, I spend much time getting to know the children, finding out what they are interested in, what they love and identifying which learning preferences suit them best. I also spend time helping children improve the intelligences/learning preferences they find challenging, so that they are better able to deal with them.

Multiple Intelligences

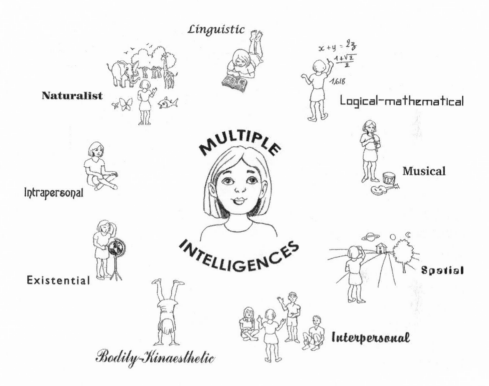

In my mind, teachers who place importance on learning styles are likely to have more engaged pupils and achieve better outcomes. It is important teachers try to strike a balance of teaching styles, so every child is reached. I also experience that, when learning preferences are accommodated, there are fewer difficulties with behaviour management in the classroom.

The following table of Multiple Intelligences and Characteristics will help you work out which intelligences your child might favour.

Multiple Intelligences	
Intelligence	**Characteristics**
Verbal / Linguistic (feel for language)	• Likes listening, reading, writing, speaking • Thinks in words rather than pictures; enjoys creative writing: poems, plays, stories; word games • Good at explaining and teaching; convincing others of their point of view • Keeps a diary/journal • Good at oral tests
Logical / Mathematical (scientific and mathematical thinking)	• Enjoys problem solving; doing experiments • Uses logic to solve problems • Likes number patterns, symbols, classifying and categorising information • Works well with flow charts; timelines • Enjoys board games and mind teasers like Sudoku
Visual /Spatial (images, art and design, 3-D)	• Likes Mind Maps®; visual organisers; use of colour • Likes pictures, collages, posters, murals • Relates to charts, graphs, maps • Enjoys videos, movies; video recording; PowerPoint slides • Enjoys constructing, fixing, designing practical objects

Musical (learning through use of pitch, tone, rhythm)	• Responds well to music • Thinks in sounds, rhythms and patterns • Plays instruments; loves singing or rapping • Enjoys composing new songs • Uses music to establish mood
Bodily Kinaesthetic (learning by doing; physical skill)	• Likes moving, hands-on activities; physical coordination • Uses body language: face or hand gestures • Enjoys modelling or crafts • Enjoys performing; role play • Enjoys food technology, design, computers, sport or art
Interpersonal (understanding and relating to other people)	• Learns through working with others; interaction • Enjoys classroom debates; pair work; group presentations; peer assessment • Brainstorms • Notices other people's mood; uses empathy; is a peacemaker • Interacts well with a mentor to guide learning
Intrapersonal (understanding yourself)	• Highly introspective and attuned to inner self: reflective; understands inner feelings • Manages own learning and in most cases is good at evaluating own performance (likes working alone)

	• Uses diaries/journals; autobiographical writing • Identifies own academic strengths and weaknesses (self-assessment) • Identifies personal goals and gives progress reports (I can...)
Naturalist (knowledge and understanding of nature)	• Likes to be outside, or enjoys outside activities such as gardening, nature walks or field trips; sitting quietly • Enjoys camping, hiking or climbing • Makes eager observations about nature • Has keen senses; observes and remembers surroundings • Shows concern for the environment, nature or animals
Existential (knowledge and curiosity about human existence)	• Asks questions about life and death • Wonders what Earth was like in the beginning • Contemplates if there is life on other planets • Ponders deeper issues e.g. human existence • Questions previous and future existence

Is dyslexia a learning style?

As you will have gathered by now, I do not see dyslexia as a disability or a condition that we need to be 'cured' of. There are millions of people with dyslexia in this wonderful world of ours who learn best using a *personalised style of learning*. I would suggest that creative learning methods should become the norm for teaching all children rather than the exception for those with dyslexia. Remember, inspiring teaching equals inspired children, which equals a greater chance of engaging in learning and, consequently, remembering information.

Dyslexia is a creative learning style

Yes, dyslexia is most definitely a learning style – the dyslexia creative learning style! The VARK (visual, auditory, read/write, kinaesthetic/tactile) model really helps to identify the many ways in which we learn; but does it consider the common characteristics of dyslexia, such as sequencing issues, language processing difficulties, disorientation, visual and auditory perceptual differences and concentration span? I believe that the concentration and attention difficulties a child with dyslexia may have in the classroom are more about *how* something is being taught and not necessarily *what* is being taught. Does your child have the same concentration difficulties when he is learning something he loves, can see the point of and finds exciting?

For me, the dyslexia style of learning is the way we learned at playschool and kindergarten: exciting learning through dramatisation, imagination, visualisation and association (DIVA). Children with dyslexia learn and communicate best by relating learning to real-life, using hands-on experience, demonstrations, experimentation, observation, visual aids, pictures, verbal communication and, above all, through being creative and having fun.

Chapter 12
Getting support for your child at school

Well, I went to college, and I spent a lot of
time there, but I flunked out many times.
I have very severe dyslexia, and so I wasn't
able to do anything having to do with much
reading. I wasn't lazy or anything.

Dr John (Jack) R. Horner, palaeontologist[60]

Many parents recommended to me for advice and coaching have arrived in tears and have been frustrated and angry that, while their child may have been recommended for some kind of learning support, few have been given regular one-to-one support lessons, or the whole process of acknowledging a learning difficulty has taken too long. For many, it has not been acknowledged at all. If fact, the ethos at one school maintained dyslexia didn't exist!

Knowledge of the educational system is vital if you want to advocate for your child. It's important to understand how the system works in your region, particularly as there seems to be insufficient funding in some schools to help all children with learning challenges adequately. In the UK, having a special educational need legally entitles your child to support in school. Because of changing governments and their policies, you need to check the latest rules for your region from your department for education.

This problem was recognised fully by the Rose Report,[61] regarded as the most important in primary education since the British National Curriculum was introduced. Government adviser Sir Jim Rose recommended that every child's reading should be monitored. Those children who need extra help should receive one-to-one support, and children with severe literacy difficulties should have the help of a specialist dyslexia teacher. Finally!

According to the report:

> Many parents reported that they have found it necessary to seek help for their child's dyslexic difficulties from outside the maintained school system. Similarly, individuals with dyslexia reported a lack of support at their schools. This chimes with a finding from the Lamb Inquiry that parents of children with SEN often say that they have to 'fight' or 'do battle' with the system to get what they need for their child.

As a parent, you are in the best position to advocate for your child. If you are in the UK, visit the UK government website (**www.gov.uk**) under Education and Learning and the Parent Partnership Service (**www.parentpartnership.org.uk**). There, you can find out about children with special educational needs.

In the USA, look at the Department for Education website (**http://idea.ed.gov**). For other countries, Google 'Special Educational Needs' and 'government education department' and the name of your region.

I believe your child should receive support the minute you or teachers suspect any learning problem. Every week you wait, your child will fall further behind at school, affecting his self-esteem, confidence and general well-being.

I think my child has a learning difficulty – action plan

It is important to liaise closely with your child's school. You may have been having an ongoing dialogue about your concerns with your child's teacher or head of year and, ideally, you will have a written record of conversations and concerns. The following plan will guide you through the process in a state school. The learning support department will initiate an assessment through your local authority. If your child is in private education, you can skip the stage of going through your education authority.

Action Plan to Get Support for Your Child

- First, **know your rights**. Read up-to-date government educational reports or white papers, so you know what your child is entitled to in terms of support and being assessed. Read the school's special educational needs policy.

- **Collect background evidence** and document your concerns that may have been raised at parents' evening, from school reports and test results, as well as any concerns about your child's emotional well-being.

- **Formal meeting.** If you feel your child's issues are not being addressed, ask for a formal meeting with his class teacher or head of year, and the head of learning support. Your aim is to gain acknowledgement from the school that there are concerns about your child's performance and well-being. Ask how teachers are differentiating work to meet your child's needs and ask for statistical comparisons for his year group regarding grades, test results and proof of progress. Teachers and learning support staff often have similar concerns to parents.

- **Support available at school.** Once a need is acknowledged and classroom differentiation is not successful, extra support either in a group or 1:1 or a qualified SEN teaching assistant or Learning Support Assistant (LSA) in the classroom should be provided. If your child has high needs, the school can ask for an assessment straightaway without going through all the formal stages of support.

- If your child is still not making sufficient progress, and you suspect a learning difficulty, ask the school for an **educational assessment**. If the school is unwilling to refer your child, I would consult the school governor in charge of special educational needs. I would also contact the Education Authority for advice.

- **Contact the Department for Education**. If your education authority has a long waiting list, or refuses to have your child assessed, then contact the Department for Education for advice or start an appeal procedure as soon as possible.

- **Independent assessment**. If all this is taking too long and you can afford it, get an independent assessment. However, you need to check with your school **before** having an independent assessment, that your school will accept the diagnosis, findings and implement the recommendations.

- **Assessment recommendations**. Once you have the assessment feedback and report, you need a follow-up meeting with the head of learning support and the head of year to agree how and when the recommendations will be put in place. These recommendations will drive the Individual Educational Plan or Learning Passport for your child.

- **An Individual Educational Plan (IEP) or Learning Passport** should be drawn up with personalised literacy, numeracy, communication, social/behavioural or study skills targets to help your child. Make sure you completely understand your child's personalised learning plan. Do not sign a learning plan unless you understand and agree with its contents.

- **Keep up-to-date with your legal entitlement** and **keep careful records** of all correspondence and meetings with all professionals at all stages of the process.

- **Try to maintain a good working relationship with teachers and the school**. When you are fighting for your child's rights, your stress levels may get the better of you at times, but remember to be polite and maintain your dignity. Most teachers want to help your child. It is generally the education/school system and funding that are a problem.

If you have been told that your child does not meet the criteria for having an assessment, I believe this does not necessarily mean he does not have special educational needs. It could mean that his needs are not severe or complex enough to meet their assessment criteria. If you are still sure that your child has a learning difficulty, listen to your gut feeling. If you can afford to, arrange a private educational assessment rather than wait or worry any longer. Prevention is better than cure, and your child should not be made to wait.

Remember, time is of the essence in helping your child catch up and not lose any more of his self-confidence and self-esteem

If you cannot afford a private assessment, there are other avenues available to you. Your local dyslexia association may offer bursaries based upon income and circumstances. Alternatively, you can discuss a referral with your doctor or paediatrician. While a dyslexia assessment is not normally covered by the health service or private health insurance, your doctor can be approached for a referral to an educational psychologist for an assessment of dyslexia if there is an illness directly related to the dyslexia, such as stress, depression or anxiety. Without a related illness, it is unlikely your doctor will be able to help.

Individual Educational Plan or Learning Passport

If your child is identified as underperforming or having a special educational need, your school should draw up an Individual Educational Plan (IEP) (or Learning Passport/Provision Map). These are teaching and learning plans specific to your child's needs, to provide support, monitor, assess and record progress. IEPs are not a statutory requirement in the UK, and many schools are abandoning them in preference for a Learning Passport, but recording and monitoring pupil intervention is lawful. They are a statutory requirement in the US.

By identifying your child's stage of learning, support can be provided to help him reach the next stage (known as scaffolding). A formal assessment will provide the background information required for the school to produce a Learning Passport or IEP, with targets for your child. This plan usually has four key areas or targets that will be addressed over a term/six-month period. The targets should be SMART (specific, measurable, achievable, realistic and time-based), and should be small steps that start with targeting gaps in your child's knowledge, then gradually building up his basic skills.

The following are some examples of targets in younger primary-school children:

- To know how to use the vowel digraph 'oa' (vowel combination to make a single vowel sound) when reading.
- To learn how to spell 25 high-frequency words.
- To join writing using clear ascenders and descenders.
- To follow and understand a sequence of events in a text.
- To use learned strategies to remember an instruction containing five parts.
- To listen carefully to instructions and not give up if it seems challenging.
- To learn the number bonds to 10.
- To practise the 2 times table regularly until automatic.

As your child progresses into secondary education, the targets will be adapted to his needs, for example:

- To use the learned letter pattern 'ough' to spell new words.
- To use connectives to link sentences and paragraphs in written work.
- To write cohesive answers to written questions based on a story, play or poem using PEE. (Point – Evidence – Explanation).
- To punctuate and set out direct speech correctly in written work.

- To organise his writing in well-structured paragraphs, using TiPToP (Time, Place, Topic, Person).
- To identify and comment on the effects of poetic language in a poem.
- To identify the maths operations required for solving 'wordy' maths problems.
- To convert fractions into their decimal and percentage equivalents.
- To proofread work following completion (for spelling, punctuation and sense).

If your child has social, communication or behavioural problems, the targets might be:

- To identify appropriate social rules and codes of conduct for various social situations.
- To work cooperatively with peers in small-group settings (e.g. share materials, allow peers to share different thoughts and take turns).
- To raise his hand and wait to be called on before talking aloud in group settings.
- To work quietly without distracting others.
- To follow routines, instructions and directions promptly.
- To complete and hand in assignments when asked.
- To demonstrate respect for others and the property of others.
- To be on time for each lesson.

Teaching interventions

There are three levels of intervention to identify and meet special educational needs in the classroom, known as the Waves of Intervention Model.

All state schools and good independent schools in England should offer a programme of Wave Intervention. **Wave 1** should be on offer in daily teaching within the classroom: the effective inclusion of all children and high-quality personalised teaching using VAK (Visual, Auditory, Kinaesthetic) teaching methods to help children with learning or behaviour difficulties.

Wave 2 should offer additional interventions to enable children to work at age-related expectations or above, typically in small groups.

Wave 3 should offer additional highly personalised 1:1 SEN interventions, for example, specifically targeted approaches for children identified as requiring special educational needs support.

Early identification is everything! The earlier the intervention, the faster your child will progress. It makes a huge difference not only in helping your child reach his educational milestones, but also to his self-confidence. If your child has slipped through the net, do not despair, it is never too late to get help. However, it may be the case your child has suffered the consequences of having low self-esteem for some time, in which case a careful course of action needs to be considered.

The earlier the intervention, the faster your child will progress

If you advocate for your child, he will hopefully get the support he needs and is legally entitled to, which will boost his self-confidence, and you will have a happier child. The children whose parents are informed and are on top of their rights are the ones who often progress the most. When your child knows that you are right behind him, he will feel supported, loved and more confident.

Chapter 13
The benefit of having an educational assessment

When I had dyslexia, they didn't diagnose it as that. It was frustrating and embarrassing. I could tell you a lot of horror stories about what you feel like on the inside.

Nolan Ryan, baseball player[62]

Early identification of a learning difficulty is paramount to our children's future and well-being.

When children struggle to remember letter sounds, or find it difficult to read, spell, write, say what they mean, or listen; process and remember information; or underperform in certain subjects; or are stressed out and overwhelmed by the learning process, of course it makes sense to find out why.

Dyslexia cannot be officially diagnosed using a screening test or a one-off assessment, but many schools in the UK routinely 'screen' young children for dyslexia, or visual stress, memory, concentration and attention, reading comprehension and vocabulary. Screening tests[63] are inexpensive and quick to administer and designed to give an 'indication' of the likelihood of dyslexia. While these tests are not a formal diagnosis, they do help teachers identify children who are at risk of a learning difficulty and who may need an educational assessment to identify specific learning difficulties such as dyslexia.

Why have an educational assessment?

If children do not find out they have a specific learning difficulty, they will not understand what is going on in their world. They will not fully get to know their strengths and challenges and will remain confused about why they are finding life at school tough. An assessment will provide you and your child with a better understanding of the areas he finds challenging, his attainment levels versus his capabilities, his strengths and learning preferences. All this information is very helpful for his metacognition.

There are several other reasons why parents decide to take their child for an educational assessment. Some feel that they do not understand fully the learning difficulties their child is experiencing. Some parents are confused, as they know that their child is intelligent and perhaps even gifted or talented in certain areas, yet not achieving academic success in school. Other parents may feel that their child's school does not understand the difficulties that he is having and is underestimating them. Occasionally, parents decide to have an assessment privately, because they simply cannot wait any longer, due to the long process of being referred by their Local Authority and feel that they need evidence to speak to their child's school with more confidence.

Whatever your reason for having an assessment, you need to be aware that it will not guarantee that your child will need or even receive additional provision in school or in external examinations. This will depend on school resources and your child's difficulties.

The British Psychological Society's Scottish Division of Educational Psychology describes an educational psychologist's assessment as follows:

> Assessment by an educational psychologist is a process which involves the gathering of information from a variety of sources in a range of settings over a period of time. It necessarily involves parents, carers, teachers, children and young people. The purpose of an educational psychology assessment is to inform future intervention. Its breadth encompasses cognitive, emotional and social factors. The ultimate aim of an effective educational psychology assessment is usually to limit the effects of barriers to learning and to promote the inclusion of the child or young person.[64]

The assessor will use norm-referenced, standardised tests that yield standardised scores, percentile rank and sometimes age-related performance. Please note that age equivalent scores are *guidelines* and should be treated with a degree of caution. Some tests use different methods of calculating these i.e. average or median, and therefore one test where a child scores 100 and gains one score based on 'average' may not be the same as another test that uses the median. Age equivalents can also have a considerable range of months either side. So it is best to refer to standardised scores and percentiles.

An assessor's report is based on thorough analysis and will provide recommendations on how parents can make the most of their child's education, as well as offering practical teaching strategies in the classroom and practical advice at home.

I would involve your school from the outset. The reasons are manifold: the assessor can obtain valuable feedback from your child's teachers and pastoral staff. With your permission, the assessor can visit the school and observe how your child participates in the classroom and playground, and generally gain a bigger picture and better understanding of your child's needs and strengths. Working together with your school will ensure a better outcome for your child.

In my experience, it is important to have your child professionally assessed to implement early intervention programmes and establish whether he qualifies for internal and external exam concessions to put him on a level playing field with his peers. Your child will not be given an easier test, but he *may* be entitled to between 10 and 25% of extra time to complete it. Your child may be offered a reader for most subjects other than English and modern foreign languages, if his reading score is below a standardised score of 85. If he does have difficulties with literacy, it may affect his ability to read all subject examinations, including maths tests (where he might be perfectly capable of doing the maths, but unable to read and understand the questions). If his speed of writing is below the average of 10 words per minute by age 11, for example, or his spelling score is below a standardised score of 85, he may be offered a scribe or be able to use a laptop in exams.

How to choose an educational assessor

If the school will not have your child assessed, and you are having to seek an independent assessment, in my view, word of mouth is generally the best recommendation – we rely on this for most things in life. Other parents will be able to tell you about someone they have used locally and with whom they got on well. They will be able to tell you whether they understood the assessment results and feedback given and whether they can recommend the specialist teacher or educational psychologist. My recommendations are to:

- ensure the assessor is experienced in assessing children with *educational* learning problems
- ask for recommendations from other parents
- check that the assessor will explain to you in lay terms the results of the assessment and recommendations
- make sure the assessor is happy and used to coming into schools, liaising with teachers and observing children in the classroom
- check that you will receive recommendations on learning strategies at home and at school and the assessor is qualified to recommend Access Arrangements[65]

If you don't know anyone who can recommend a specialist teacher or educational psychologist (Ed. Psych.), you can go on to your country's psychological testing centre website, where you can search by region. In the **Appendix**, I have listed websites where you can find assessors, educational psychologists and speech and language therapists in many countries.

What is assessed?

Before an assessment takes place, the assessor will want to know how successful your child feels as a learner and how this affects his overall motivation to learn. In preparation, you should receive a family questionnaire about your child's development.

Typical Contents of a Family Questionnaire

Medical history: any problems during pregnancy or at birth; allergies, problems with nutrition, illnesses, dates of last hearing and eyesight tests

Family background: family members with reading, writing, spelling, numeracy or attention difficulties, for example

Developmental history: achieving normal milestones and any difficulties

Educational history: schools attended and any gaps in education

Strengths and talents: what your child loves and is good at

Learning issues: what you perceive the learning difficulties to be

Emotional issues: relating to self-esteem and self-worth

Sensory or physical issues: motor coordination skills, physical or sensory difficulties

Social, behavioural or communication issues: friendship problems, attitude to peers and adults, behaviour in school and at home

With your permission, another questionnaire should be sent to the school to obtain complete information about your child's development and performance in school. The assessor is interested in finding out where your child is positioned in relation to the rest of the class in academic subjects, particularly English, maths and science.

To gain a holistic understanding of your child's abilities and strengths, I always want to know about a child's performance in non-academic subjects such as art, sports, technology, drama and music, as well as any extra-curricular activities he enjoys. These are often areas where your child may excel. This kind of information really helps me understand the whole child and serves as positive reinforcement of his strengths. It is also invaluable information for building up his self-esteem.

The assessor will also need information about any special needs provision your child is already receiving and whether he has an IEP/Learning Passport or a 504 plan (USA) and what his IEP targets are. The assessor will also be interested in your child's own perspective on many aspects of his life in and out of school.

Typical Contents of a School Questionnaire
• Overall ability • Attainment levels and assessment results in all subjects • Behaviour and contribution in the classroom • Attitude to work, adults and peers • Friendships • Self-esteem and motivation • Any other specific concerns teachers may have

After considering all the background information and feedback received from the parents and teachers, the assessor will select several tests (see table of Battery of Tests). The assessment itself usually takes a few hours to conduct, using formalised tests as well as observation.

Selection (Battery) of Tests
• Verbal comprehension • Visual perceptual reasoning skills • Working memory: auditory and visual • Processing speed • Visual–spatial awareness • Gross and fine motor skills • Phonemic awareness and sounds knowledge • Reading ability and comprehension • Writing ability and speed • Spelling ability

- Arithmetic and maths ability
- Organising and planning ability
- Metacognitive skills (how he learns best)
- Social, communication and behavioural skills

When should a child be assessed?

The hereditary origin of dyslexia makes it possible to identify children at risk early on so, as soon as you suspect a learning difficulty, particularly if there is a hereditary link, have your child assessed. Or, if you realise that your child is not making sufficient progress on Wave 1, 2 or 3 (class differentiation, group intervention or specialist 1:1 teaching), seriously consider having an assessment.

In an ideal scenario, I recommend an initial assessment at age 7/8 to identify the extent of your child's learning difficulties. However, as many children's learning difficulties may not have been identified until they reach secondary school, the first assessment may well take place when your child is around 11 years. In secondary or senior school, an up-to-date assessment is required by examining boards to qualify for exam concessions in formal examinations such as GCSEs, iGCSEs, A-levels and the International Baccalaureate (IB).

If your child is in the private sector in the British educational system, he will also need an up-to-date assessment before sitting Common Entrance at 12/13 years of age.

So it's a good idea to plan ahead for when assessments might be needed and get the timing right.

Once in higher education (college or university), youngsters will need another updated report to qualify for the Disabled Students' Allowance (DSA) in England or Student Awards in Scotland. This allowance is available to all teenagers and adults who meet the criteria. They may qualify for a laptop, software, hardware, training on the new equipment they receive, a photocopying allowance and some learning support. So it is well worth spending the extra money (again) on updating their assessment!

In the USA, modifications in graduation requirements for students with disabilities vary from state to state: some states offer no modifications, but the overall trend nationally is to allow for some modification of graduation requirements for students with disabilities who might not otherwise graduate.[66]

If your child is granted exam concessions, he must be given plenty of time to practise using this extra resource within exam conditions as it takes time and much practice for children to learn how to use these unfamiliar resources.

Assessment results

The result of the assessment is a unique 'profile' of your child's ability – a unique pattern of his strengths and weaknesses, individual test results (with standardised scores, percentile rank and sometimes age-related performance), a diagnosis of a learning difficulty, if there is one, and recommendations.

A full confidential report is usually produced within 3–4 weeks and it should include the following recommendations:

- Suggested ways forward in supporting your child
- Focused programmes or therapies to promote successful learning
- How to play to your child's strengths
- Exam concessions/Access arrangements (reasonable adjustments): for example, the possibility of extra time or using a scribe, reader or technology in tests and examinations
- Ways to raise self-esteem
- Study skills, revision and memory skills suggestions
- If required, a referral to an occupational therapist, speech and language therapist, eye or ear specialist or paediatrician for further investigation.

A report may be up to 20 pages long and is bound to contain some unfamiliar terminology or concepts, but the assessor should review and explain the outcomes with you. I like to summarise the key scores on one page to make it easier for both parents and teachers to read and digest at a glance.

A summary of the key findings and recommendations should be distributed to all subject teachers, teaching assistants, learning support and pastoral staff, so that everyone is working together to provide the best support for your child.

No assessment is complete until the recommendations are implemented, both at home and at school

I believe that no assessment is complete until the recommendations are implemented into your child's daily life, both at home and at school. Parents play a vital role in the whole process: before, during and after the assessment. Teachers should feedback to all staff about any academic, social, emotional or behavioural implications and provide training where neccessary. In my experience, the child achieves greater success when both the school and parents implement the recommendations and work together.

Parents are often keen to know their child's Full Scale IQ, but the individual scores of the subtests in each of the four categories below, plus the strategies a child uses, provide excellent in-depth information about your child's specific areas of expertise and difficulty. The same applies to understanding the strategies a child uses in the attainment tests.

The Full Scale Intelligence Quotient (FSIQ) is made up of the average of the four scores below. The General Ability IQ (GAI) is the average of only two first scores: the VCI and PRI. You will find definitions in the **Glossary**.

- Verbal Comprehension Index (VCI)
- Perceptual Reasoning Index (PRI)
- Working Memory Index (WMI)
- Processing Speed Index (PSI)

Sometimes, the Full Scale IQ cannot be interpreted, because of an unusual set of results. This is why the test results need to be interpreted by their individual scores so that strengths and weaknesses can be identified, which will enable the assessor to suggest strategies to overcome any weaknesses and play to your child's strengths.

The Full Scale IQ and General Ability Index scores are important academically, as they indicate your child's ability to achieve and thrive in an academic environment. While working memory and processing speed are not indicators of general intelligence (i.e. verbal comprehension and non-verbal reasoning), they are clear indicators of how easily your child can process, remember and recall information. Therefore, generally, a child with a lower or average Full Scale IQ and learning difficulties will find a highly academic environment extremely challenging.

A child with a high Full Scale IQ who is diagnosed with learning difficulties may excel in many areas but struggle with some aspects of learning. This is recognised in the UK as 'dual or multiple exceptionality' (DME), and these children who have 'high learning potential' also have one or more special educational needs (SEN).

It can be very difficult to identify dual or multiple exceptionality, as the child's difficulties can be masked by his high learning ability. In other words, if the child's difficulties were addressed, he would be achieving much higher results.

In the UK, a standardised score of 130 and above represents 2% of the population who are 'gifted' or 'very able'. However, you need to know which test was used to assess your child for the scores to be meaningful. On the British Mensa website (**www.mensa.org.uk**), there are guidelines and minimum test scores to rate a child's intelligence and giftedness.

There are a variety of IQ tests that may be used to test your child's intelligence, each with its own scoring system. For example, a top 2% standardised score in any of the frequently used tests below qualifies your child (over 10 years of age) for entry to Mensa,[67] should you wish to register:

Cattell III B	– 148
Raven's Advanced Matrices	– 135
Wechsler Scales	– 132
Culture Fair	– 132
Raven's Standard Matrices	– 131

Every school should have a 'high learning potential' or 'gifted and talented' (G&T or GAT) register, which is a list of children whose learning needs are unlikely to be met without specific planning and differentiated provision.

If you believe that your child falls into this category, ask your child's school for its eligibility criteria. These are guidelines only; the decision is generally based upon checklists, assessment scores, standardised tests, teacher nominations, parent information, observation and even peer nomination.

Knowing your child's level of giftedness or learning potential should ensure that he does not underperform or become bored in the classroom. I believe that parents are the best people to know whether their child is gifted or talented. Such children need to be identified so that their intellectual, social and emotional development can be managed well. How this should be done, however, depends on the age of the child, and whether he is happy or presenting problems to parents and/or in school.

Explaining the assessment and results to your child

It is important to explain carefully and lovingly to your child, in language that he will understand, why he is having an assessment. Children are very perceptive and will generally sense that something is going on, and you most certainly do not want him to worry endlessly about things that may be incorrect or that he fears might happen.

Most parents are able to gauge the best way to let their child know what is going to happen. It depends on how sensitive your child is about his learning problems, and his level of maturity.

For very young children, parents may not want to make a big deal about the tests, and may gently explain that the tests are fun and are to find out what he enjoys doing and is really good at. But for older children, we owe it to them to be honest. By honest, I do not mean being blunt or unkind about why they are having an assessment, or saying they are having a dyslexia assessment (as they might not even have dyslexia) or even explaining the tests in too much detail. But you could explain a little about what they involve, that the tests will identify which learning preferences they have, where their strengths lie and establish why they are finding things tough, and that having this knowledge will help them learn more easily.

You need to discuss the report recommendations with your child, otherwise he may assume the worst. If any of us undergo any test and the results are not discussed with us, we worry endlessly about the outcome.

Remember that children's development stages are dynamic, and that the assessment results will change after a number of years, which is why educational boards and universities require updated assessments. Sometimes, with good, early intervention and coping strategies, your child may cease to need exam concessions or a particular method of intervention. We also see that, with good intervention and the right student motivation, some scores can improve over time.

If you do discover your child has dyslexia, he is likely to go through what I call the *five stages of accepting having dyslexia*. Whenever we suffer a dramatic shock in our lives, psychologists have agreed that we undergo five stages of grief. For example, the loss of a loved one or a divorce can lead to the five stages of denial, anger, bargaining, sadness and acceptance.

From my experience, many children go through five similar stages of accepting having dyslexia. I also witness many parents going through similar stages of fear and anger when they find out that their child has a learning problem. Parents also need guidance from professionals, so that they understand, feel supported and empowered to deal with this lifelong journey in the right way.

In order to help our children, we need to be armed with the right information about dyslexia: its positive attributes and guidance about what having dyslexia means. Take a look at the following table of The Five Stages of Accepting Having Dyslexia.

The Five Stages of Accepting Having Dyslexia

Stage 1 – Relief: Depending on your child's age and personality, the first stage of discovering that he has dyslexia may be relief. Very young learners are often relieved to discover that they are not silly, but in fact part of a very large group of the population; and, despite finding certain aspects of learning in school difficult, they are smart.

Or

Stage 2 – Denial: Some children will not initially accept that there is anything holding them back. They enter into denial about being 'different' from their peers: 'There's nothing wrong with me!' In their heart, no child wants to be different from their friends. If learning support is offered, they may refuse it or rebel against it.

Stage 3 – Anger and resentment: Once the initial diagnosis has had time to sink in, they may feel angry and unable to direct their feelings. Why me, it's not fair? Why do I find reading or spelling or writing stories so hard? I am smart and good at many things, but why can't I do as well in school as my friends?

Stage 4 – Sadness or depression: Some children may develop intense feelings of sorrow or pain and negative thoughts about their abilities and find it difficult to talk about how sad they feel. They may become more active or misbehave to cover up the painful feelings. We need to watch out for the symptoms of low self-esteem or depression.

Stage 5 – Acceptance: Children embrace help. They discover their learning preference, strengths, develop their talents and begin to use and understand different learning strategies to manage their weaknesses. We teach them how to be self-confident and believe in themselves. They learn to understand that they have a huge amount to offer the world. Children become optimistic about their future.

The support and reassurance you provide for your child is very similar for all the phases: it is important to allow sufficient time for your child to come to terms with having dyslexia; and then sensitively reassure your child, focusing on all the positive aspects of dyslexia and the extra support he will receive.

Some people are against the idea of 'labelling' a child as 'having dyslexia'. If people with dyslexia had been given a different name, way back when it was first identified, and we had been called 'holistic thinkers' or 'dynamic visualisers', then we wouldn't bat an eyelid at being associated with such a positive label. However, I have come to the conclusion that, at school, identification is critical in ensuring that our children receive the support and care they need in order to thrive at school and in the wider world.

What happens after an assessment?

Having an educational assessment is just one part of the whole journey on your child's Road to Success. Unless the recommendations are put into place both at home and at school, then what is the point of having the assessment done?

If dyslexia or any other learning difficulty is diagnosed, it needs to be carefully managed. Make sure one person is responsible for coordinating and ensuring all recommendations are put into place and that all teachers are made aware of your child's strengths and challenges. If your child does not have an IEP/Learning Passport, then one should be drawn up straightaway, with specific measurable targets to help him make progress; and he should, of course, have learning support.

I believe the benefits of having an educational assessment go way beyond the advantages of improving learning at school. Knowing our strengths (and challenges) as adults will guide us to make better decisions in our choice of further education, college or university course, adult career and the jobs we choose for the rest of our life.

Chapter 14
Choosing the right school

'Dyslexia was an embarrassment at school.
At ten, I still had problems reading and
writing.
And children can be cruel when they
discover that you are different.'

Sir Steve Redgrave, Olympic gold medallist[68]

As parents of children and teenagers with learning difficulties and special educational needs, we not only deal with the constant challenges in our everyday life, we also face the pressure of making sure that our child benefits to the full from the education system.

Many parents come to me feeling quite overwhelmed about the best way forward, particularly given the differing and even conflicting advice they receive from their local authority. So it is no wonder that parents are unsure how to go about choosing the right school for their child.

Depending on where you live and your catchment area, most children with mild to moderate learning difficulties can be taught through mainstream education provided the school has excellent provision for regular one-to-one support, or dedicated classroom assistants. Some schools have 'dyslexia-friendly' status, which makes it easier for parents to narrow down the choices. In some parts of the country, parents simply do not have enough choice because of catchment area issues.

If your child has moderate to severe learning needs, physical or sensory impairments, or any other complex need that may affect his schooling, you may have to look at a specialist SEN school or come out of state education, as not all state schools provide adequately for children with dyslexia -

which is absolutely outrageous. Consequently, some parents consider homeschooling or sending their child to a private school. Some private (independent) schools have excellent provision for dyslexic learners, but they may not always advertise this.

Considering a specialist SEN school or a private school maybe a daunting prospect financially, socially and morally. If you find yourself having to go down the specialist school route, you need to find out exactly what your child's requirements are, and that is another reason for having an educational assessment, so that you know what you are dealing with. The better you understand your child's learning problems and his abilities and talents, the greater the chances of choosing the right school.

Finding a school

Finding the right school for your child involves research. It is important to do your homework thoroughly before visiting or selecting a school. Word of mouth can be a great recommendation but, if you are new to an area or your friends' children have different requirements, there are several organisations online and books written about how to choose and find a good school.

In the **Appendix**, I have listed many organisations across the world where you can begin your research. Browse several school websites, review the school prospectus for any additional information about entry requirements, special educational needs and extra-curricular activities. I would also ask for a copy of the school's SEND/Inclusion policy and the school's inspection report (performed by OfSTED or the Independent Schools Inspectorate in England). Check out what the report says about SEND provision in the school, pastoral care and extra-curricular activities.

Unfortunately, the SEND policy is a rather lengthy, sometimes confusing, document for the non-specialist to wade through and understand fully. The key things to look for in this document are the school's procedures for undertaking an assessment and the timescale taken to identify and assess learning difficulties (if your child has not already been assessed). You also need to find out the number of lessons per week that are offered to pupils with SEND and whether your child will be offered group or one-to-one support.

The timescale taken to identify your child's needs and obtain support is vital. The process of carrying out a statutory assessment by the local authority can sometimes take far too long. Being told your child will be assessed 'as early as possible' is not specific enough. You need to know how soon, when and how often your child will receive support before he attends that school.

When you are happy that you have all the information you need, contact a few schools and book an appointment to visit. Ask for meetings with the Headteacher and the Learning Support Department, so you can gauge the school's attitude to special needs and understand the provisions it makes.

Visiting schools

Visiting a school is always the best way to get a 'feel' for it: by seeing the facilities, observing the teaching and seeing a whole school in action. You will be able to gauge the Head's enthusiasm and attitude to 'every child matters' and whether he is confident and interested in interacting with the pupils and teachers. You will be able to see if the classrooms look cheerful and fun, take a look at pupils' work on display and see whether it seems appropriate for their age. You will also be able to see whether the teachers are fun and interactive with pupils, and the pupils' reaction to the teachers. You can observe pupils' behaviour in the classroom and during break time.

Notice boards provide a quick and easy way to find out what types of activities are going on outside the classrooms and can lead you to ask questions about extra-curricular activities such as drama, art, music and language clubs.

Make sure you talk to lots of pupils about what they love about the school and what they're not so keen on. Even take a look in the dining room and at the menu to see what is on offer. You can tell a lot from this about how much variety and care has gone into selecting a good school menu.

Selecting a New School

- Do all subject teachers use multisensory (visual, auditory and kinaesthetic) methods?
- Are children's multiple intelligences taken into consideration when planning a lesson?
- How is teaching adapted to meet the needs of Wave 1 in the classroom? Does the school individualise teaching to the needs of each child within the classroom? Ask to see a class in action.
- What is its process for identifying Wave 2 and 3 or intervention?
- How large are the classes? Children with learning difficulties need smaller class sizes to get the attention they need.
- What learning support or teaching assistance is available in the classroom?
- Does the school have high expectations for pupils with dyslexia or other learning difficulties? Can the school give examples of pupils' success?
- What provision is made for 'high learning potential' or 'gifted and talented' children?
- Is there a special needs learning support specialist? If so, what are his or her qualifications? Are there enough learning support teachers in the school?
- How many times a week are one-to-one lessons provided? How many pupils are in each group for group support?
- What remedial programmes do they use?
- From which lessons are children removed for support?
- How much homework do children get?
- If your child needs speech and language therapy or an occupational therapist, can the school organise someone to come into school?

- What kinds of support or resources does the school offer parents?
- Does the school view non-academic subjects as being just as important as academic subjects?
- What pastoral care is in place to support pupils with academic, social, emotional or behavioural difficulties?
- What sort of enrichment activities does the school provide? This is important so your child can develop his talents in sport, drama, music, dance, design, woodwork, cookery, art, textiles, technology, debating skills or any other exciting activities.

Most importantly, make sure you have your list of questions at the ready, and make notes to refer back to.

I would also ask to speak with a few subject teachers who will be teaching your child, to ensure they are all working from the same principles. You will be able to gauge a lot from this.

Does the school have high expectations for pupils with dyslexia or other learning difficulties?

You will also need to be ready to answer questions about your child. Armed with your child's educational psychologist's report, and feedback from, say, his current school, sporting, music or drama coach, for example, plus your own experiences within the home, you can present a learning profile of your child: his strengths and weaknesses, his interests and activities and his personality. That way both the school and you will know whether the school is right for you and your child.

My advice would be not to choose a school just because it says it offers provision for dyslexia or learning difficulties. Choose a school because it suits your child and offers additional activities to develop his particular interest or talent, and excellent pastoral care.

However, if you cannot find the right school or you need help choosing between a couple of schools, an educational psychologist or an educational consultant can offer you good advice about the suitability of schools locally and further afield.

Concerns about your current school

If you are at all concerned about your child's progress, your child is unhappy or his behaviour has deteriorated, ask for a meeting with relevant staff members as soon as possible. You should never have to wait until the end of term to be told that your child is underperforming or unhappy, or that his behaviour has deteriorated. The school can provide you with regular updates about your child's progress, in the form of:

- Individual standardised tests, such as reading, spelling, maths, verbal and non-verbal reasoning tests or any other ability and achievement information
- Curriculum-based assessments
- Classroom-based assessments
- Work samples of your child's progress or lack of progress
- Individual Educational Plan
- Mid-term and end-of-term reports
- Parent interviews with subject teachers, including non-academic subjects such as sports, performing arts, music, technology or design.

All teachers (class or subject teachers) should fully understand your child's challenges and strengths and be able to explain to you what allowances are being made in the classroom and how they are differentiating the teaching to accommodate your child's personal needs.

Establish a good relationship with teachers

This is essential. I strongly encourage keeping an open dialogue with your child's teachers. With smaller children, it might be easier to accomplish in person, whereas older children will feel embarrassed if mum or dad keep showing up at school. Your teacher can give you valuable insight into how your child is really doing in class, how he interacts with other children and where he trips up on work tasks. The teacher can also help you make sure that homework assignments are properly understood.

Teachers' workloads are generally very heavy, with most teachers still working after school hours in their free time, so I would limit communication to a couple of times a week. You can write a short message in your child's homework diary and a short email is a really great way of maintaining communication, and allows teachers to respond when they have a minute. It also provides a record for everyone to refer back to.

PART FIVE
Supporting Your Child's Learning

Chapter 15
Learning challenges and solutions at school and home

I know what a dyslexic child goes through – the frustration of not being able to do what other children do easily, the humiliation of being thought not too bright, when such is not the case at all... Accept the fact that you have a problem. Refuse to feel sorry for yourself. Realise you don't have an excuse - you have a challenge. Never quit!

Nelson Rockefeller, 41st Vice President of USA[69]

In order for learning to take place effectively, children's hearts and minds must be stress-free. Children with dyslexia learn best when they are in a non-threatening environment and can take their time, be creative and learn through hands-on personalised experiences. They need to feel good about themselves, free from worry, and able to concentrate fully in the classroom. To be ready for learning, children must be emotionally, physically and mentally prepared for it.

Children with dyslexia learn best when their learning is personalised, and they are in a non-threatening environment

Children with dyslexia display many, many strengths in the classroom, including:

verbal reasoning	creative and artistic ability
non-verbal reasoning	emotional intelligence
oral and debating skills	generating ideas

| general knowledge | problem solving |
| visual–spatial awareness | leadership |

Apart from the obvious challenges of reading, comprehension, writing, speaking or spelling, there are other challenges that are less easy to detect but which can impact learning quite significantly nonetheless. For example, their ability to maintain concentration, process information or commit to memory may vary significantly from their verbal or visual strengths.

Self-esteem and behaviour

Self-esteem is a massive concern for dyslexic learners, especially in the classroom. How does your child feel if he is underperforming? Not good, I would suggest. The result of low self-esteem may impact on his behaviour.

The way in which a child behaves reflects to a large degree what is going on inside. A child who is frustrated and confused by his learning environment or overwhelmed by his learning challenges may act out his frustration in various ways. He may be aggressive, angry or rude, or act as the class joker, sitting in the back row disrupting the class behind the teacher's back by making funny comments, passing notes and so on. Or, he may just withdraw.

How does your child feel if he is underperforming?

Bad behaviour and attitude often reflect feelings of low self-esteem. Children who mess around in the classroom may be experiencing learning difficulty, but the reverse may also be true. Sometimes bright children who are not sufficiently challenged by their class material act up, tune out or otherwise make life difficult for the teacher.

There will be times when it will be very hard to discipline your child, especially once you understand dyslexia, and what your child experiences because of it. Your child needs boundaries in the same way that all children do. He needs to know that you will catch him when he falls, and correct him when he wanders off in the wrong direction.

Absenteeism

A child with poor self-image or learning difficulties is likely to be absent from school more often than other children. If you discover that your child is arriving late to lessons or playing truant, it's a sign of not being comfortable in the classroom. Try to find out if there is one particular class he tries to avoid and why he dislikes it so much. Perhaps he has not done the home-work or has trouble relating to the teacher or the material?

If you are inclined to allow your child days off for 'not feeling well', try to find out the exact nature of your child's resistance to school that day and see if there is something you can do to help (or ask a teacher for help) rather than letting him take the day off. The problem only gets worse, as he not only misses vital information, but has the added stress of having to catch up.

Friendships

Emotionally healthy children form friendships with peers who are most like them, usually in their own class or age group. Sometimes unusual friendships develop between older and younger children. This might be perfectly natural if the two are in a club together outside school or their families know each other, but it can also be a sign that things are not quite right.

An older child who regularly associates with younger children might be experiencing low self-esteem and difficulty fitting in with his own peer group. Likewise, a younger child who regularly seeks out the companionship of older children might be experiencing feelings of insecurity or lack of self-confidence with children his own age. It may not be significant, depending on the circumstances, but is something to be aware of.

Check your child's relationship with his peers is healthy and that he is not being put down or bullied by anyone. If you ever suspect bullying, act on it right away. A child who feels emotionally or physically threatened will be distracted from learning and will feel low.

The most important thing is to take time to listen to your child, let him vent his frustration and do not dismiss his feelings because, in the moment of frustration, the feelings are very real and the difficulties seem insurmountable. Things will be all right because the two of you can work together to give him coping strategies and successful techniques for dealing with his feelings.

Likewise, a child who is exhibiting symptoms such as irritability, unreasonableness and anger towards siblings is probably dealing with a great deal of internal turmoil. It is important to talk calmly with your child to understand the underlying cause of the stress. Do not make assumptions or write it off as personality. It could be because of learning difficulties or because something else is going on.

Organisation

Some dyslexic learners can find it overwhelming to tackle large projects or ones that have many components. One way to help them overcome this is to break the project into smaller, manageable pieces (known as chunking). This approach works for everyone, but is particularly helpful for people with dyslexia.

When my daughter had to clean her room all she could see in her untidy room was one big mess. She didn't know where to start, would look around and be overcome by the myriad details involved in cleaning even a small part.

Help your child get organised

To overcome the feeling of the impossible, start with a small statement such as, 'Start by making your bed', then explain the steps for making the bed:

> 'Take any items that are on the bed and put them on the floor.
> Pull up the covers over the bed.
> Smooth them out.
> Arrange the pillow neatly at the head of the bed.'

These are simple steps a child can follow and will help your child feel less overwhelmed. Once the bed is made, identify the next task.

> 'Now go and pick up all the dirty clothes off the floor, and everywhere else, and put them in this laundry basket.'

Break projects into smaller, manageable pieces (chunking)

This technique of small steps works well with all manner of projects, including homework and general life management tasks. In time, your child will learn to break things into tasks by himself and unravel the complexity of any project so that it is made up of small, manageable tasks.

One important tool to help organise children who have dyslexia is the ability to prepare things in advance. We cannot prepare for every possible occasion, but there are many times when being organised will go a long way to preventing your child from feeling overwhelmed.

Stress and coping

Children with learning difficulties are likely to suffer stress at times when a teacher decides to give a spontaneous test or quiz, or calls on students to read a passage aloud or make a presentation in class. Speaking in public, for some people, can be stressful – many non-dyslexic people have a serious dislike of public speaking. Imagine how it must feel to a child struggling with reading?

Dyslexic learners need extra time to prepare for tasks such as reading and writing assignments and tests. It can be frustrating when a well-meaning teacher who had a spelling test planned for a particular day suddenly has to adapt a lesson plan and move the test to another day. Your child, who may have spent hours studying for the test and got himself into a state, now feels he wasted his time and, because he finds it difficult to remember, will have to start all over again in preparation for the test on another day.

Learning to roll with the punches is not easy for any of us and can be especially tough for those children who are trying hard to keep their grades up. Anger takes its toll on us emotionally and saps energy we need for other things. Rather than try to brush the episode aside and make it sound as though it doesn't matter, give it due attention. Letting your child air his feelings on the subject in the short term will help him get back on track in the longer term. At the same time, he will be learning coping strategies that will give him tools to deal with other frustrations as they come along.

Self-confidence comes from a feeling of adequacy and being able to cope

Self-confidence comes from a feeling of adequacy and being able to cope. If we have coping strategies for specific situations handy in the front of our minds, it is easier to handle difficult situations when they arise. Having coping strategies at the ready is especially important for people with dyslexia.

Peer pressure and bullying

Some of the biggest challenges to your child at school may come from other children. Kids can be brutal and don't always realise the impact their teasing can have. Two things are going on here that are difficult to overcome. Children are naturally sensitive and self-conscious.

Young adolescents can seem overly preoccupied with how they look physically, and become self-conscious about every last hair out of place. They also become very sensitive about personality quirks or any little thing that other kids at school will pick on. Even the seemingly perfect child will imagine that he has innumerable defects and that everyone in the world will notice how inadequate he is at this or that. This is a normal phase of adolescence. However, being subjected to an inordinate amount of teasing at this stage can leave indelible scars on our hearts and our egos.

There is not much you can do about other people's children, but you can certainly talk about it with your own child. Discuss the fact that some teasing is normal. Invite your child to listen in with new ears on what kids are saying to other kids and ask them to imagine what it must feel like.

The point is to deflect attention away from themselves and help them to develop a thicker skin by understanding that they are not necessarily being singled out (although it may feel that way) but are simply being subjected to the same sort of teenage teasing we all go through. However, if the teasing is on-going and nasty, that is bullying and is not acceptable.

Metacognition – self-aware learning

We learn best when we understand how we learn and take an active role in setting ourselves up for success by employing techniques that we know fit best with our personal learning preference. The process of exercising control over your own learning is called 'metacognitive learning'. It means that we are aware of how we learn, which allows us to stop and think about what we want to learn, so that we can apply the best technique. For example, if we know that copying a poem on to a separate piece of paper and highlighting key words helps us to memorise it, then that's the approach we should take.

Another aspect of metacognitive learning is self-monitoring. This means that, if we read a passage, we then need to measure how well we have understood it. After a reading assignment, your child can ask himself a series of questions (perhaps you can help) to see if he has absorbed its meaning. If he has not understood, then he needs to take action, such as re-reading, summarising or visualising the passage or making notes.

You can teach your child to be a metacognitive learner by asking what works and does not work for him. For example, he may realise that he gets better results with his homework when he works on a full stomach, so he may decide to save homework until after the family meal.

When your child takes charge of his own learning, he will decide for himself to ask for help when he needs it, but this is a level of maturity that you will need to help him attain.

A metacognitive approach to learning is a useful tool for all children, but especially for a child with dyslexia. In order to use it effectively, you need to understand what learning styles work best for you and apply those learning preferences in your approach.

Memory and over-learning

Children with dyslexia learn best when teaching is structured, targets more than one learning style and revisits and reviews previous learning. A common characteristic of dyslexia is the difficulty to organise information in the brain in a linear manner. When information is fed to the mind in a variety of ways and reviewed frequently, it forms many different pathways in the brain and has more chance of filtering into long-term memory and circumventing the organisational problems from which dyslexic learners suffer.

Variety is also important when trying to assimilate information from a dull history topic or to master spelling.

Over-learning = practise = automaticity

When we hear the same information over and over, it becomes familiar. New information needs to be repeated more than once. When we make some kind of association with the new information, it is much easier for us to remember.

Concentration

When your child loses concentration or hits a roadblock and can't seem to master the spelling of a word or the point of the story, stop and let him take a break, get up and move about, or turn to an easier subject for a mental break. Come back to the topic with a positive attitude. Inspire your child to keep at it by reminding him he overcame another problem successfully through perseverance.

My child won't accept help

What do you do when your child does not accept the fact that he could benefit from help at school or at home? Many parents have to face the immense frustration that their child will not accept help or has a complete lack of motivation.

In most cases, children do not want to be different from their peers, but a lack of motivation may be due to several other things, ranging from anxiety, depression or fear of failure to the end goal seeming unattainable. Sometimes, children do not know how or where to start or it all seems like too much hard work for no reward. Occasionally, children are disaffected because of everything they have been through.

Most people do things either because they love doing them or because they fear the consequences. When children or adults have a dream they want to pursue or a goal they want to achieve, they are more inspired and motivated to be successful. This is where you come in. Try and find out what his goals are (short and long-term), what he feels he needs to do or become better at in order to achieve those goals; and ask him what support you and teachers can give him.

Motivation and reward

The human psyche, while complex on many levels, is based on a very simple model. Everything we do is underpinned by a single unconscious principle: we move away from pain and towards pleasure. If pain and pleasure exist in equal measure in a single objective, we are more likely to give up the pleasure and walk away from the pain than we are to move towards the pain in order to experience the pleasure. This leads us to a natural conclusion about human motivation: in order to get people to do things, you have to reduce the pain and increase the pleasure. Relating motivation to learning, you can prepare children to have an open heart for learning by:

- making learning fun – be creative
- breaking down difficult learning tasks into easier, more manageable, ones
- finding tricks and tips that work to overcome learning difficulties
- reducing any stress induced by learning difficult material
- reducing barriers and roadblocks to learning
- offering incentives for achievement and reaching goals

To keep motivation high, always focus on the positive and do not dwell on the negative. Use the following motivational techniques to encourage your child:

- Help your child define his goal (**he** needs to identify and define his goal)
- Start small: break the goal into manageable pieces (use a motivation chart)
- Set personal rewards for achieving each mini goal

- Practise/revise consistently, but don't overdo it
- Include doing something fun or in a fun way
- Allow your child to learn from failure
- Encourage your child to evaluate his progress and celebrate success
- Positive reinforcement
- Reward effort

It is better to set a series of small, short-term learning goals with small incentives ('Let's get your maths homework finished up, then I'll make you a nice cup of hot chocolate and you can watch your favourite TV programme'), than offering large incentives for longer-term goals that may seem impossible to reach ('If you can read this whole book in a week, and write a 500-word essay on it, I'll buy you that new video game'.) The video game may be a greater incentive but, if the goal is perceived as too difficult or unattainable, it will serve only to discourage your child and make the work seem harder than ever. You can use big incentives for long-term goals as a special prize for reaching multiple short-term goals. In other words, break the problem down into small, attainable chunks.

The best way to monitor progress and motivate your child is to have a reward motivation scheme in place. It should be a simple chart that you set up and agree to with your child. Your child needs to 'buy' into it, therefore, he needs to be involved in setting it up. Use fun pictures that he has chosen, e.g. his favourite football team, a humorous picture. Then have a weekly schedule where he ticks off or inserts smiley faces when he has done his task. State what the task is: 15 minutes of practising phonics sounds, reading or times tables every day. State what the reward is: for example, after 5 smiley faces I will get some stickers or chocolate or get to choose what we do at the weekend; after 20 smiley faces I get to buy my favourite comic or book. After 100 smiley faces I will get a new video game.

If you have tried the 'softly, softly' approach to motivating your child and it is not working, some tough love is in order. You may need to take away privileges in a way that will encourage your child to earn them back. I would still work through the motivational techniques, so that he knows where he is heading, how he is going to get there, and what the reward is at the end (either personal reward or privileges returned). Take a look at the **motivation charts** in the Appendix.

Whole-school approach

As our understanding of dyslexia and other learning difficulties continues to grow in the UK and other countries, it is becoming apparent that techniques that work for children with learning challenges also work really well for children who do not suffer from those 'disorders'. Studies and research originally intended to help dyslexic learners are benefiting the whole school.

A whole-school approach to multisensory learning and using multiple intelligences means teaching all children, not just special needs children, using multisensory (using many of the senses) techniques. If you have a specialist educational report, you will have a good idea of the challenges that your child faces, and also the challenges that the teacher faces. I encourage you to have an open relationship with your child's teachers, and not to be afraid to let them know what does and does not work for your child. It is not easy for a teacher to identify the specific learning challenges of each child in his or her care without a diagnostic educational report.

If your child regularly has difficulty with a particular subject, for example, find out from the teacher which teaching strategies he is using and discuss ways to help your child learn more effectively. Knowing a child's learning preference and teaching to his preference will improve his chances of learning the material. Perhaps your child could have one-on-one teaching to explain a difficult concept or topic?

Dyslexia challenges and solutions in and out of the classroom

The following tables give many of the challenges that children with dyslexia may experience in and out of the classroom, and I have offered solutions.

Dyslexia Challenges and Solutions In and Out of the Classroom	
Self-esteem	
Challenge	**Solution**
Feelings of inadequacy	Praise as much as possible and remind your child of all the things he is good at. Complete the table **Identifying Your Child's Talents and Gifts** to focus him on everything he loves doing. It will make him feel better about himself.
Low grades	Help your child revise, by suggesting the right tools, appropriate environment and motivation techniques at home for studying. Celebrate effort and any improvement.
Withdrawal from lessons for support makes your child feel self-conscious and unhappy	Explain having 1:1 help can provide significant gain and feelings of support. It is important your child is not taken out of core subjects, as he cannot afford to miss out on new topics. It is also important not to be taken out of his favourite subject or break times – these lessons provide relief and may be an opportunity for him to excel. Your child needs break times to relax and restore his energy levels: he needs exercise and needs to play, interact with peers and maintain his friendships. Timetabling support lessons within school can be complex; so lessons before or after school or doing extra practice at home is good – 15 minutes every day using specific remedial programmes.

Can't understand new concepts	Explain using real objects, role play or using analogies.
	Ask your child to explain back the concept to check understanding.
Not enough positive feedback	Positive feedback is essential both at school and at home, every day, several times a day.
	Give encouraging feedback and offer positive solutions; do not assume your child has the skills to do this alone.
Revises, but can't remember facts	If information is not being retained, review how revision is being done. Just reading through class notes will not help him remember facts he learned several months ago.
	When we revise, we try to make facts memorable, summarise and review each topic using Mind Maps®, mnemonics, memory links, pictures, colour, highlighting, rhymes, music, role play etc.
Oversensitive to criticism Teacher highlights too many errors	Congratulate your child for attempting and producing work.
	Use friendly-language that identifies specific errors and focuses on 1 or 2 key areas: grammar or punctuation or spelling or style – not everything all at once.
	Get a template of what the work should look like.
Wants to be as good as his friends	Make sure your child finds his unique quality and excels at something. Help him find his special talent.

Behaviour and Social Skills	
Challenge	**Solution**
Absenteeism	If your child misses a day at school, he has the stressful task of catching up with work and his peers. If he gets too far behind, he will end up taking more time off due to stress starting a downward spiral.
	Make sure your child gets catch-up work for all subjects missed – help him catch up.
	Discover the route of the problem.
Immature or bad behaviour	Poor behaviour can be attention seeking and may be in part due to low self-esteem or lack of understanding.
	Look at ways to boost your child's confidence and talk to him kindly when you catch him behaving badly.
Peer pressure	Teach your child that independent thinking and responsible behaviour and knowing right from wrong are the best approach.
Class joker Disruptive	Acting the clown is usually due to low self-confidence or the need for positive attention.
	Can he do the work? Is he bored?
	Make sure your child is getting enough of the right kind of attention in the classroom or break time.
	Check he is happy. Then work on strategies to boost self-confidence.
Seen, or sees himself, as less clever	Talk to your child about dyslexia not being linked to lack of intelligence – it is a difference in learning. Relate to friends who have overcome it and

	what strategies they used. Point out what he is good at and encourage him to pursue those activities inside or outside school. Ask a learning support teacher for help.
Exhausted Can't sleep well Too much going on at school or home	Make sure your child does not spend longer than required doing homework. Is your child worried about something? Is he getting enough time to relax at home, burn off energy or get to bed on time? Stop stimulating activities at least 2 hours before bedtime (i.e. computer games, TV, any electronic equipment). Limit extra-curricular activities after school to a couple of times per week, especially if there are homework commitments.
Aggressive Anti-social behaviour	Aggression is a big sign of low self-esteem and struggling with learning difficulties or other symptoms of growing up. Check for depression. It is vital to find the source of the anger. Most schools run behaviour or support groups within school. In complex situations, seek help from a child therapist to support the child at home and at school.
Withdraws Tearful	If your child seems depressed, talk to a school counsellor or your doctor.
Avoids working	Even when the teacher has explained what needs to be done, your child

	might not have the confidence that he will get it right and still doesn't understand what to do. If your child is young, talk to his teacher and let him know the problem.
	If your child is older, suggest he has a quiet word with the teacher himself, or send an email on his behalf.
	Is your child bored because he finds the work too easy? Check he is doing work that is challenging him.
	Let his teachers know how your child is feeling.
Can't explain feelings	For young children, using Teddy Bear cards with different facial expressions can help them identify how they are feeling.
	For older children, encourage them to talk to a best buddy or let them know that you (or the school nurse / counsellor) are there for them when they are ready to talk.
Stressed out

Anxious

Difficulty coping

Overwhelmed by volume of tasks | Involve the teacher. |
	Reassure your child that everything is going to be OK – and you are there to help. Your child will instantly feel supported and less stressed out.
	Help him prioritise work: get your child to write down in a diary everything he needs to do.
	Get him to write down the completion date, subject, title plus 3 bullet points for what needs to be done for each assignment.
	Show your child how to gather information, put it in order and prioritise.

Environment	
Challenge	**Solution**
Room temperature	Make sure that the room is neither too hot nor too cold. Boys often prefer a lower temperature than girls.
Acoustics Background noise	Acoustics are important for dyslexic learners with auditory processing difficulties, as they often struggle to differentiate sounds in words, in particular, the endings of words. Background noise or echoes can be a problem. If the acoustics are not right, ask the teacher to sit your child at the front of the classroom. Sit away from the window and chatty children.
Lighting	Flickering lights, fluorescent lights or poorly lit rooms will disadvantage most children, but particularly those with learning difficulties who may be easily distracted or affected by sensory problems. Report problems to the school.
Uncomfortable chairs	Check that your child's chair is at the right height to write at the desk comfortably, so that his back or neck does not hurt and his feet are touching the ground.

Auditory and Listening Skills	
Challenge	**Solution**
Can't remember instructions	Short instructions are best – maximum 3. Then increase slowly to 4, then 5.

Auditory processing difficulty Difficulty processing spoken word	Ask for colour-coded instructions to be written and left on the board or have a printed list next to your child's desk. He needs to sit near the front of the class so he can focus. Encourage your child to keep a small notepad in his pencil case to jot down reminders using symbols/mnemonics to help him remember certain tasks he has to do every day, such as the layout of a new writing task: Write the <u>D</u>ate on the right, <u>U</u>nderline it, then <u>M</u>iss a line and write the <u>T</u>itle, <u>U</u>nderline it, <u>M</u>iss a line and <u>S</u>tart writing = DUMTUMS. Ask for handouts. Ask the teacher to check regularly that your child understands the task. If problems persist, have an auditory processing assessment.

Visual Skills	
Challenge	**Solution**
Visual processing problems	Up to 10% of all children in the classroom suffer from undetected visual problems. If your child has a routine eye test and does not need glasses, but is still complaining about words blurring or 'sliding off the page' or is suffering from headaches, visit a Behavioural Optometrist.
Loses his place when reading	Use a finger under the text to keep place.

Black print on white paper causes glare	Try using a coloured overlay plastic ruler/A4 sheet. Print on coloured paper.
Can't copy accurately from the board or text book	Sit near to the front of the class. Joined up handwriting might be difficult to read on the whiteboard; ask the teacher to print writing and write in lowercase. Ask for handouts for anything more than a few sentences.
Long- or short-sighted	All teachers need to be made aware if your child has to wear glasses for certain tasks. Ask the form tutor or class teacher to notify all staff.

Attention and Concentration	
Challenge	**Solution**
Can't concentrate for long periods Daydreams	Ask to sit near the front of the classroom to help him focus better. Ask the teacher to help him stay on task.
Fidgety Needs to move about	Varied activities that focus on all learning preferences, especially bodily kinaesthetic, are best. Fetching a drink of water, handing out work or changing tasks involves moving around. Stress balls help reduce fidgeting, but you need to be careful that your child does not switch off from doing school work while fidgeting with a ball.

Memory	
Challenge	**Solution**
Leaves homework or equipment at school or home	Ask for homework to be handed out at the beginning of the lesson, written in the school homework diary and checked. Ask the teacher to check all the necessary books are put straight into his school bag.
	Ensure your child puts homework back into his schoolbag as soon as it is done.
	Set up a memory board at home where he can check which activities he has to prepare for: swimming, sports kit, homework to hand in and so forth.
Forgets the time	Use a memory jogger (set a watch alarm) to remind your child if he has to be somewhere for an extra music lesson, etc.
	Write down all the days/times he has special lessons and keep it in his pencil case or school diary. Let the teacher know.
Loses clothes or possessions	Label all clothes and possessions. Use a permanent marker pen or sew-on labels (iron-on labels come off).
Forgets messages	Write messages down for your child so he can deliver them without having to worry whether he may forget the contents.
Can't remember timetable	Photocopy the timetable, drawing symbols to represent each subject, and keep it in the front of your child's school diary.
	Keep a copy at home on his notice board.

| Difficulty remembering phoneme sounds | Practising phonics regularly is essential for reading and spelling.

Use a phonics programme at home for 10 minutes a day to build up knowledge through repetition and practice. |

Organisation	
Challenge	**Solution**
Forgets to bring right equipment to lessons	Get your child into the habit of making lists using diaries and calendars. Prepare a list of equipment required for each subject. Encourage him to use a transparent pencil case to see at a glance what is missing.
Files not in order Can't find things Disorganised or over-organised Messy schoolbag Messy locker	Show your child how to organise his files and folders by using file dividers and a contents page. Number the pages and list a contents page for your child to find information more easily. If files are organised well, your child will feel less confused. Periodically, children need help reorganising equipment and putting books/files into order. It is much easier to start doing this with help, rather than on one's own. Show him how to do it for future reference. Being over-organised can also have its drawbacks. If your child is obsessed with being overly organised, it may distract him from doing the work. Check that your child is getting the work done.

Organising ideas Planning work Settling down to work	Dyslexic learners may need much help organising ideas and putting them in order. Sit with your child and ask questions to prompt his thinking, and get him to plot his ideas into a Mind Map® or linear list (if he prefers) before he starts writing. Use the outline to double-check that all the important headings and sub-headings are discussed.
Presented with too much written information	Too much information creates brain overload. Information is best presented in manageable chunks. Show your child how to separate it into smaller sections with headings. Highlight important information and jot down a heading/title/picture next to it.

Reading	
Challenge	**Solution**
Difficulty tracking left to right Words on page appear blurred or 'move around'	Black print on a white background can make reading 'uncomfortable'. Try using a coloured overlay plastic ruler to stop glare or words 'moving around' and help keep one's place. There are many different coloured overlays, but the yellow or blue ones tend to be the most commonly used. Print on cream-coloured paper.
Print is too small, difficult font to read	Font size minimum 14 pitch, sans (without) serif, e.g. Comic Sans, Century Gothic or Arial.

Omits/inserts words Loses his place	Suggest putting his finger under the words when reading, or using a plastic reading ruler.
Hates reading aloud	Ask teachers not to select your child for reading aloud, if he feels embarrassed.
Difficulty decoding	Practise decoding skills using a remedial decoding programme.

Comprehension	
Challenge	**Solution**
Difficulty interpreting what is said	Check that meaning has been understood, ask for an explanation and clarify in simpler language.
Misunderstands questions	Double-check understanding of the question. Check all question words can be read correctly (who, how, why, what, when, where, which, etc.) Often there is confusion between 'who' and 'how'.
Can't remember what has been read	If decoding is a problem, check understanding after a few sentences. If your child is reading too fast, try to practise reading more slowly and for meaning. Ask your child to draw a symbol or picture next to a paragraph to jog his memory. Discuss text content. Then ask him to visualise the whole story and make a pretend video in his mind.

Speech and Language	
Challenge	**Solution**
Difficulty explaining what he means or expressing ideas verbally	Encourage your child to recap or summarise texts after reading small sections. Be patient if your child struggles for words. Use pictures to express words or meaning. If problems persist, have a Speech and Language assessment.
Lack of exciting vocabulary	The best way to boost vocabulary is by reading or listening to audio books. Encourage reading by choosing topics your child loves. Read books that are not too advanced and with age-appropriate interest, with large, dyslexia-friendly text and lots of pictures – even for older children. Play synonym games.
Speech impediment	A speech therapist can treat an impediment by retraining the muscles of the mouth, jaw and throat to work together.
Literal understanding	Try and not use innuendos or double meanings; if you do, explain what they mean.
Difficulty answering 'open' questions	Open-ended questions that address cause and effect may be difficult to answer. Use questions that require only a one-word or one-sentence answer. Multiple choice questions are easier to answer.

Handwriting	
Challenge	**Solution**
Slow handwriting speed Writing causes fingers, hand, arm, shoulder or neck to ache Poor body posture Wriggles in seat while writing Complains of headaches Incorrect placement of writing on a page Slanted away from the margin Writes above, below or through the line Inconsistent letter formation	Teach body and spatial awareness, correct body posture and tripod pencil grip before attempting to correct handwriting problems. <u>Check pencil grip</u> Is he holding the pencil correctly in the tripod grip? Is he gripping the pencil too tightly? Is he pressing too hard on the paper? Is his hand twisted awkwardly? Recommend using a soft pencil grip; triangular pencils or Lamy-style pens with three indentations for correct placement of fingers. Paper should be angled at 30° to the left for right-handers or 30° to the right for left-handers. <u>Check seating posture</u> Back should be straight into the chair. He should not be sitting on his knees while writing. Check his legs are not swinging under the desk – if they are, the chair is too high. Is he supporting his head with his hand? Is he wriggling in his chair while writing? Does he prefer to stand up at the desk to write? Does his mouth move while he is writing? If your child is exhibiting several of the above symptoms, he would benefit

	from seeing an Occupational Therapist who specialises in handwriting.
Handwriting not joined up

Incorrect letter formation | Use Handwriting Without Tears[70] paper, Handwriting for Windows[71] or equivalent with double lines to teach your child how to place letters.

Practise cursive handwriting using a remedial writing programme. Ask for a copy of the school writing programme to practise at home.

Attend handwriting club in school. |
| Reverses letters b–d | Prepare a memory card with a picture of a bed and the word to show b/d direction. Form a 'b' and 'd' by forming a circle and touching your forefinger and thumb together on both hands, keeping the rest of your fingers vertical to make a 'b' with your left hand and a 'd' with your right. |

Coordination Skills	
Challenge	**Solution**
Gross motor control issues	Exercises such as balancing, wobble board, climbing, hopping, skipping, dribbling a ball, catching a ball or beanbag, sport or martial arts.
Fine motor control issues	Exercises such as tracing, dot-to-dot, tracking, cutting, painting, modelling, doing puzzles, threading beads, rolling and picking up marbles or sticks, creating card towers or sewing.

If your child has fine motor control issues, it is best to address any gross motor control problems first. If problems persist, visit an Occupational Therapist. |

Writing and Spelling	
Challenge	**Solution**
Written tasks take too long	Allow extra time.
	Ask for differentiated tasks: gap-fill exercises to minimise writing.
	Give writing cues and templates.
	Reorganise written paragraphs into correct sequences: this helps with logical sequencing as well as being a model for the task.
	Scribe for him. Older children can learn how to touch-type and use a laptop.
Slow note-taking	Teach abbreviation and note-taking techniques. Use a recording device.
Difficulties expressing thoughts in writing	Get your child to express thoughts verbally at first. Then, sketch ideas on a Mind Map® before any writing takes place. Use story-writing templates and cues.
Forgets learned spellings	Practise spellings in word families where possible.
Inconsistent spelling or grammar	Use trace, copy, cover, write with your eyes shut template and target all learning preferences. Colour code or use mnemonics. Learn high-frequency spellings. **www.icanspell.co.uk**.
	Use a handheld Franklin Spellchecker[72] and Thesaurus to check spelling and find synonyms for adjectives and adverbs.
	Ginger Software[73] checks grammar and spelling according to the context of the text – excellent for dyslexic learners. Practise literacy skills with e.g. Wordshark[74].

Maths	
Challenge	**Solution**
Difficulty remembering times tables	Ideally, your child needs to aim for automatic recall out of order, if he is to be able to do mental arithmetic and calculations without a calculator. Regular practice every day and repetition, and teaching to learning preference, is the only way to remember the times tables. Use fun games: card games, CDs, free interactive games or numeracy software such as Numbershark.[75]
Can't remember sequences of a calculation, maths rules or specific formulae	Use mnemonics (memory links). For example: to learn the Circumference of a Circle equation – use the expression 'Cherry Pie Delicious' which corresponds to C=Pi x Diameter. Pi is a commonly used term in maths: Pi = 3.1416 (rounded to 4 decimal places). To remember the sequence of numbers, we use the sentence 'May I have a number', where the number of letters in each word relates to the Pi number (May = 3, I = 1, Have = 4, A = 1, Number = 6).
Can't understand wordy maths problems	Does your child have difficulty reading? If so, read the question out to your child. Then ask him to write numbers or maths symbols above the word so that the calculation becomes easier to see. For multi parts to a maths question, highlight different calculations in different colours, and show each step on a separate line.

Can't remember meaning of maths vocabulary	Put maths words on flash cards with their meaning and the symbol on the reverse. Keep them in a pencil case for easy referral. Write difficult words on flash cards and practise linking word to meaning using games such as Happy Families, Pairs or Snap.
Can't remember number bonds to 10 or 20	On flash cards write 0 on one side and 10 on the back, and the same for 1 and 9, 2 and 8, 3 and 7, 4 and 6, 5 and 5. Put large dots on each side of the flash card so that your child can count them if need be. Colour-code them. You can even turn the numbers into rhymes or associate animals with each number. Let the child choose the colour and the animal, as he will make a connection and remember it better. Play fun card games with them. Do the same with number bonds to 20.
Reverses/ transposes numbers when writing	Practise tracing over difficult numbers using a mini whiteboard with dotted numbers and arrows to show direction of number.
Transposes numbers when reading	If your child puts his finger under each number as he says it, he is less likely to read 12 for 21. Or get him to imagine a T U (tens and units) written above the number.

Sequencing	
Challenge	**Solution**
Story ideas	Use a story plan template with pictures. Verbalise a plan and plot/draw the ideas before writing.

	Provide a selection of key nouns, verbs, adverbs and adjectives.
Times tables	Give your child a foldable plastic times tables square to keep in his pencil case. Practise fun learning techniques.
Maths calculations	Give a visual summary of maths procedures and examples to refer back to, e.g. BIDMAS (Brackets, Indices, Division, Multiplications, Addition, Subtraction).
Days of week, months, seasons	Play board games, card games, musical CDs.

Directions and Orientation	
Challenge	**Solution**
Differentiating left and right	The left hand held up makes an 'L'. Play games, such as Simon Says or Hokey Pokey.
North, East, South, West	Use mnemonics: Naughty Elephants Squirt Water
Reading maps	Use maps with picture cues.

Time Management	
Challenge	**Solution**
Can't tell the time	Clock faces are complicated for dyslexic learners. It is best to learn analogue even though digital is easier.
	Make a clock face with swivelling hands, ask your child to draw in the 1-12 numbers and write 'past' and 'to' either side - e.g. 5 past next to the 1, 10

	past next to the 2 etc. Play time games. Wear an analogue watch.
Concept of time	Some dyslexic children find the concept of time and today, yesterday, tomorrow, past or future quite tricky. Have conversations with your child about what you did yesterday, what you are doing today or tomorrow and link it to the past or the future.
Not enough time to finish work in class	Children who work hard in class but are unable to finish their work should not be punished by having to finish it at home alongside homework. Speak to the teacher to understand what is causing your child not to complete the work in the class.

Homework and Revision	
Challenge	**Solution**
Takes long time to complete	If your child takes longer than the recommended time per subject, don't allow him to do more. Let the teacher know there is a problem. Or if your child wants to finish an important project, give him a hand, note how long it took, and inform his teacher.
Doesn't always understand what is expected Incoherent notes	Check that your child has brought home all the books he needs. If he hasn't written down the homework correctly, check the homework assignment on the school internet portal. Ask for homework handouts that explain everything that needs to be

	done, so that you can help your child if necessary.
Difficulty prioritising	Put a planner (calendar) on the kitchen wall of when assignments and homework are due using pictures. Or use a school diary and highlight in red the homework that needs to be handed in first.
	Check whether any research needs to be conducted, as this should be started as soon as possible, even if the hand-in date seems far ahead.
Difficulty revising for tests or exams	Suggest study skills lessons at school or teach your child how to revise at home. Draw up a revision plan and suggest your child revises one subject at a time. Buy cheap, new revision exercise books for each subject. This way pieces of revision paper are not lost, and the book can be kept for future revision of the same topic. Demonstrate how to use Mind Maps®, index cards and flash cards. Display difficult revision material on a notice board, where it can be regularly seen.
	Encourage your child to drink water when revising. Every 15 minutes take a water break and a brisk walk round the garden or house and take in some fresh air. Water and oxygen fuel our brains.

Good teaching is one-fourth preparation
and three-fourths theatre.
Gail Godwin[76]

Chapter 16
Literacy skills and tips

I hated school... One of the reasons was a
learning disability, dyslexia, which no one
understood at the time. I still can't spell,
because I see some of the letters backwards.

Loretta Young, actor[77]

Reading, spelling, handwriting, writing or speaking are five of the most common areas that trigger us to sit up and take notice that dyslexia might be in play. These areas cause some of the most common frustrations that many people with dyslexia face to one degree or another.

With early detection and intervention, many people with dyslexia are able to work around and otherwise overcome the debilitating effects of poor reading and spelling skills. Others, usually those whose condition is never sufficiently addressed, do not learn to read effectively, and suffer the lifelong effects of poor self-esteem, lack of coping skills and not realising their potential.

I am writing this book because it doesn't have to be that way! With structured help, most children with dyslexia can go on to higher education if they want to and have fulfilling careers. It is possible, with hard work, to learn to read and to spell. It requires a lot of patience and teaching methods that are designed for multisensory learning (using more than our eyes and ears for reading). It requires teaching and acquiring coping skills and persistence, for both teacher and pupil.

There are many reading, spelling and handwriting remedial programmes that teachers and parents can use. Certain resources may not suit some children so bear this in mind. I use a wide variety and select the best resource according to a child's learning preference, specific challenge and personality.

Because the effects of dyslexia vary widely from one individual to another, I urge you to talk frequently with your child about what method is working, what he is seeing, hearing and experiencing, as well as what styles of learning he seems to enjoy most. It is very discouraging to be the one spending hours catching up or 'staying behind' to get homework completed. It is frustrating enough having the 'condition' without being subjected to all kinds of tortuous techniques for overcoming it. Above all, I encourage you to make the whole experience fun – whatever that takes and whatever that means to you and your child – rather than a painful ordeal that neither of you wants to face every night at homework time.

Putting yourself in your child's shoes

If you don't have dyslexia, it can be difficult to appreciate what a dyslexic learner experiences. One misconception is that dyslexic learners confuse 'b' for 'd' or 'p' for 'q' because they do not see the letters correctly. Some do experience blurred or wavy vision. Others may see perfectly normally but have tracking issues; some have trouble *remembering* whether the 'b' or the 'd' has the stick to the right or the left. Try to find out which it is for your child. What letters, what sounds, what groups of sounds present difficulty and exactly what kind of difficulty do they present?

A technique I recommend for you as the teacher/parent to help you understand how your child feels is to practise reading and writing backwards, upside down or in the mirror, similar to the way Leonardo da Vinci wrote. Another way to get a feel for how dyslexic learners feel is to read a page of, say, Greek or Russian or any unfamiliar foreign language. Even as a competent linguist of European languages, trying to remember the letter sound correspondences of these two languages blows my mind. Now you can begin to appreciate what your child is experiencing.

Use plenty of teaching aids, especially visual ones such as pictures, hand gestures, and even common household products, to help your child learn how to read. Remember the golden rule of dyslexic teaching, which we have mentioned before but it bears repeating (no pun intended!):

Repetition, repetition, repetition

Remember also to keep teaching sessions short, take breaks, have fun, get comfortable and don't worry too much about mistakes.

Despite the fact that English is one of the most widely-spoken languages, it is not easy to learn, especially from the perspective of reading. English spelling is not always phonetic and is largely inconsistent. No sooner do you master a sound and how to read it, than you discover that there are multiple ways to spell that sound and multiple ways to pronounce it.

Consider the words 'read' and 'wind'. Did you pronounce those in your mind as 'reed' and 'whined' or 'red' and 'winned'? What about the following words:

pair	their	wear	red	by
pear	there	were	read	bye
pare	they're	where	reed	buy

Those are just a few simple examples. How did you learn these words? Think back. You probably used a lot of rote memorisation. There are rules to English and these can be learned and applied. However, there are almost as many exceptions as there are rules and patterns and these also have to be memorised. Memorising spelling rules is a complete nightmare for a dyslexic learner!

Learning how to read

Pre-reading skills

- **Rhyming skills** (an important precursor to reading, and one that many children with dyslexia find difficult)
- **Matching** (patterns, shapes, letters and words)
- **Motivation** (being excited and interested about books)
- **Visual-motor skills** (tracking from left to right)

- **Print awareness** (how to handle a book, noticing that the print has a function, and that each word on a page represents a spoken word)

- **Narrative skills** (being able to describe things and retell a story)

Rhyming and alliteration are important skills when it comes to reading (and for language development, social skills, writing and spelling too).

It is a common trait among people with dyslexia to find discriminating between certain sounds difficult, in particular the endings of words. Since rhymes generally depend on the sounds at the end of words, dyslexic learners sometimes have trouble telling the difference. At the same time, words such as 'fit' and 'fat' do not sound significantly different from each other, making it hard to process, and ultimately remember the difference between them.

So, if your child is still young enough to enjoy nursery rhymes or poems, it will help your child if you emphasise the last word of each sentence as you sing or recite together. Then you could ask your child to think of other words that rhyme with the endings of the rhymes and turn it into a fun competition.

Reading skills

Depending on the age of your child and current ability, the following areas will help develop reading skills:

- **Phonemic awareness** (the ability to notice, think about and work with individual sounds in a word)

- **Phonological awareness** (phonics – letter sounds: a method to teach how to sound out words)

- **High-frequency words** (about 150 most commonly-used words that cannot be easily decoded using phonics; plus about 120 medium-frequency words)

- **Vocabulary** (understanding the meaning of the word)

- **Fluency** (tone, whether you read smoothly or choppily, using punctuation and intonation)

- **Comprehension** (understanding what is being read).

Phonemic awareness

Phonemic awareness and phonics are not the same. Phonemic awareness is the ability to notice, think about and work with individual sounds (phonemes) in a word, and understand that words are made up of smaller sounds.

Many children with learning difficulties find it tremendously difficult to process phonological information and learn how to relate letters of the alphabet to the sounds of language. For all children, the processes of phonological awareness and phonemic awareness must be systematically taught. When children learn nursery rhymes, they are playing with sounds and experimenting with language. When they read funny books such as Dr Seuss's *Cat in the Hat*, they are using what they have learned so far to extend their phonological awareness and improve their reading skills.

Phonological awareness: Phonics – letter sounds

Many dyslexic learners are visual learners and, because they often find remembering phonics difficult, may revert to whole-word learning. The problem with this is that, when children are learning how to read, it is difficult to memorise every single word in the English language, plus they don't acquire the skills needed to sound out complex words.

Teaching reading using phonics means teaching the sounds that are associated with letters individually and when combined together. This can make a big difference in children's ability to read, spell and comprehend the written and spoken language.

A word is broken down into syllables and units of sound (phonemes). You should first learn each phoneme before you can break words down into syllables. There are approximately 44 sounds in the English language and sometimes the same sound is spelled differently, but being able to distinguish the sound is vital to being able to master its spelling. Once you identify the sound, you then have to apply spelling rules and choose graphemes (a letter or sequence of letters that represents a phoneme).

There are approximately 44 sounds in the English language, not 26

If children are hungry to learn how to read before they go to school, then you can start by teaching them to read the first 45 high-frequency words by sight. Alternatively, start them off with a phonics programme, to ensure that they are learning the units of sound correctly. When phonics is taught in a fun, playful, multisensory, repetitive manner, it is not a laborious task for our kids. When children are young, they learn through play and having fun – the more fun and creative it is, the more their hearts and minds are open to learning and remembering.

Most schools teach synthetic phonics, which is a structured system of teaching reading by first teaching the letter sounds and then building up to blending these sounds together to pronounce the whole word. Children are taught segmentation skills by hearing the sounds within a word and blending skills by merging these sounds together. For example, to read the words 'thin' or 'farm', we don't sound out each letter 't-h-i-n' or 'f-a-r-m'. The correct way to read the word is to sound out and blend each phoneme: 'th-i-n' and 'f-ar-m'.

For some children with dyslexia, learning synthetic phonics can be a nightmare! Children with dyslexia may find it easier to work with slightly larger chunks of a word. For example, instead of sounding out 'b-a-t' as individual phonemes, sounding it out as 'b-at'. (known as Onset and Rime). A multisensory approach is definitely the most successful way to learn phonics, and teaching it on a 1:1 basis often gets good results.

I shan't go through the whole process of presenting the letter sounds and the order in which they are learned – as there are structured programmes that do that. But the table of 44 Phonics Sounds will give you an idea; I have put a word next to the sound to help you create the correct sound.

There are 20 vowel phonemes, which are notoriously trickier to learn than the consonant phonemes. So, when helping your child learn vowel phonemes, I find it helps to present words together in word families that have similar sounds and patterns. Such as f-**igh**-t, l-**igh**-t, m-**igh**-t, n-**igh**-t, s-**igh**-t and t-**igh**-t. Colour-code them on to flash cards and play happy families or snap.

44 Phonic Sounds

Consonant phonemes

1. /b/ – bat	13. /s/ – sun
2. /k/ – cat	14. /t/ – tap
3. /d/ – dog	15. /v/ – van
4. /f/ – fan	16. /w/ – wig
5. /g/ – go	17. /y/ – yes
6. /h/ – hen	18. /z/ – zip
7. /j/ – jet	19. /sh/ – shop
8. /l/ – leg	20. /ch/ – chip
9. /m/ – map	21. /th/ – thin
10. /n/ – net	22. /th/ – then
11. /p/ – pen	23. /ng/ – ring
12. /r/ – rat	24. /zh/ – vision

Vowel phonemes

1. /a/ – ant	12. /ow/ – cow
2. /e/ – egg	13. /oi/ – coin
3. /i/ – in	14. /ar/ – farm
4. /o/ – on	15. /or/ – for
5. /u/ – up	16. /ur/ – hurt
6. /ai/ – rain	17. /air/ – hair
7. /ee/ – feet	18. /ear/ – dear
8. /igh/ – night	19. /ure/ – sure
9. /oa/ – boat	20. /ə/ – farmer
10. /oo/ – boot	(the 'schwa' /ə/ – is an
11. /oo/ – look	unstressed vowel that sounds similar to /u/)

Here's a handy little rhyme for you to remember some of the long vowel combinations: /ai/, /oa/...

> When two vowels go walking,
> the first one does the talking.
> First vowel, long vowel, say your name.

The silent magic 'e' or bossy 'e' has the ability to change short vowel sounds into long ones. For example:

m**a**d becomes m**a**d**e**;
h**o**p becomes h**o**p**e**;
c**u**b becomes c**u**b**e**.

High-frequency words (sight words)

Even though there has been much debate about whole-word learning versus synthetic phonics, there is much utility in the approach of whole-word learning when it comes to learning the 250–300 high- and medium-frequency words, also known as 'sight words' (or Dolch or Fry words).

**The first 100 high-frequency words account
for more than 50% of EVERYTHING we read!
Learn them by heart.**

It is easier for dyslexic learners to memorise these common words by heart and consequently learn to recognise them by sight. They can be found on **www.icanspell.co.uk** or **www.carolinafrohlich.co.uk**.

Did you know that the first 100 most common words account for more than 50% of EVERYTHING we read? If your child can learn these by heart, it will significantly speed up his ability to read and spell. Take a look at the spelling section in this chapter for how to memorise high-frequency spellings.

Vocabulary

Vocabulary refers to words and their meanings. Reading is the best way to build vocabulary. Other ways include watching documentaries, and being curious enough to ask the meaning of words when you hear unfamiliar ones. Another good way is to use an online thesaurus when writing assignments. For example, when you read over an essay, look up alternative words if you find you have used the same word many times.

To work on vocabulary with your child, point out common roots for different words and discuss their origin or meaning. For example, 'phono' means sound, hence the words phoneme, microphone, telephone, phonetic and so on.

Fluency

Fluency in reading (writing and speaking) can be likened to automaticity. When we are first learning something, we are slow to perform and have to stop to think about things. Certainly, a five-year-old reader will not (usually) read as rapidly as a ten- or fifteen-year-old.

Repeating the same task often makes it familiar and the action of performing it is moved to another part of the brain that makes good use of our long-term memory. The task becomes more automatic.

Reading, writing, listening and speaking are just like any other tasks. The more we do them, the more automatic they become. The more we read, the more we recognise common words and, as we continue to exercise our reading skills, we begin to recognise less-common words. This relates to vocabulary building as well. Reading fluently is then only slightly interrupted by coming across a word we have never read before.

Comprehension

It is quite common for children with decoding problems not to understand what they have read. Their brains are concentrating so hard on segmenting words into syllables, decoding units of sound and blending them all together that, by the time they have got to the end of the sentence, they have often forgotten what they have read.

Some children may have decoding difficulties but good comprehension skills, and are still able to get the gist of what they are reading by remembering key words and thereby verbally answering comprehension questions accurately.

I have also come across children with very good decoding skills and a good level of reading accuracy who do not comprehend fully what they are reading. This can be quite confusing for parents, but remember that every dyslexic learner is different, and no two children have exactly the same learning problems.

Whatever their challenge, it is important always to use questioning techniques and discuss, after each paragraph or section, what your child is reading. If need be, draw a little sketch or symbol next to the paragraph to summarise the content. This way, if he is reading a comprehension passage, for example, he will be able to glance back immediately at the pictures and visualise and remember the whole story.

Higher-order thinking skills for reading and comprehending

Higher-Order Thinking, or HOT, is a technique used both to improve and challenge learning such as reading and comprehension. It includes techniques such as asking questions, summarising, visualising and predicting outcomes. You can infer something once you know something else, make a connection from one thing to another and predict an outcome based on something you already know. Studies have shown that using HOT techniques with children in basic literacy teaching[78] greatly enhances their ability in reading comprehension.

HOT is similar to metacognitive awareness because it requires awareness and the use of thinking skills as one reads. The immediate goal is to improve understanding of what is being read, which in turn leads to greater learning.

Higher-Order Thinking gets students more engaged in the text and, as that happens, they are more likely to understand it. This is particularly helpful for dyslexic learners, who can sometimes be so focused on reading individual words that they fail to make the overarching connections in the storyline.

It is a common complaint among dyslexic readers that they do not get as much out of a book as non-dyslexic readers. Here are the principle HOT techniques and how they help children learn.

Questioning

Questioning can be something readers do by themselves or at the guidance of a teacher or parent, who may direct children as follows:

Ask yourself questions about what you have just read and what it means (both literally and in the context of the story). If a character is performing an action you don't understand, ask yourself why? Perhaps you missed something earlier in the text or perhaps the author is setting up the plot and you are not supposed to know the answer yet. Either way, asking questions can help to keep you alert because you will be looking for the answers to the questions, and thinking about new questions as you read on.

Making connections

The teacher leads readers through a series of prompts or questions to draw connections between what they are reading and their own lives, a situation in a movie they have seen or another book they have read, using graphs, pictures or charts, or simply talking about it.

Visualising

Visualisation means creating an image in your mind of what is going on in the text. Doing this forces you to concentrate on what you are reading. Constructing a scene, a building or a character in your mind's eye from the words on the page helps to identify the action, remember it, and draw from it for some of the other techniques, such as predicting and making connections.

Predicting

If you follow the story and are picking up on foreshadowing (authors' hints), clues, characters' personalities and so on, it becomes possible to make predictions of future plot developments. How will a character behave when he finds out what someone else just did? The predictions may or may not turn out to be accurate but the point is to be following what is going on in the plot and thinking ahead.

Inferring

Inferring essentially means reading between the lines. The author may be explicit about what is going on but may leave readers to draw their own conclusions.

Predicting and inferring are closely related; each helps you do the other. Make notes about what you inferred or predicted and then, as you read on, verify if you were right. Note-taking can be formal, with a dedicated notebook to jot down ideas as you read, or it can be informal, such as using sticky notes and placing them in the pages of the book as you go along.

Summarising

The ability to summarise a passage, a page or two, or an entire chapter reinforces what you have learned and helps you determine what was important in what you have just read.

Summarising is a useful skill to learn in general and, in the context of reading, it helps you clarify the essential elements of the story. If a book summary or a literature essay is required after reading the book, write down the summary points for each chapter as you go along. This will provide a basis for the essay and a written document to jog your memory.

As you summarise, think about the main points of the story, significant events, and the actions of peripheral characters as well as those of the main characters. What is the author trying to say? If your child is uncomfortable summarising in writing, ask him if it would be easier to draw pictures or symbols.

All this may seem like a lot of trouble for reading a book, and takes a long time. However, over time it will become easier and more intuitive, and your child will learn to do it alone. That is the real benefit that you are after: the ability to set your child up for success when teachers and parents are not there to help. So have patience with this technique, go slowly at first and rest assured that your child will reap big benefits in the long term.

Learning how to spell

Teaching spelling (encoding) is similar to, and the reverse of, teaching reading (decoding). Phonemic awareness and spelling go hand in hand. In order to be able to spell, it is important to be able to identify individual sounds within words. Once you have understood that certain combinations of letters make certain sounds, then you extend the concept to understand that certain sounds are formed by certain combinations of letters.

Spelling can be much harder than reading for dyslexic learners because, when two different groups of letters make the same sound (such as 'maid' and 'made'), it is easier to recognise the pattern visually than it is to remember which one to use when writing. The fact that 'made' and 'maid' have the same pronunciation is a difficult concept to teach, and it is more difficult to remember which grapheme (letters or groups of letters in written language) to use when you have to spell the word for yourself. This is one of the reasons that dyslexic learners may have poor spelling skills and often spell words phonetically.

Both parents and teachers are bewildered by the fact that a child may be able to memorise spellings for a spelling test and perhaps get them all correct, but go on to misspell the same word frequently in extended writing. The odds are that your child has learned his spelling list quickly, revising the day before, and using a strategy that is not suitable for him in the long term.

Of course, there are several spelling schemes available, and remedial programmes that your school will be using. So I am just going to give you some tips and techniques that I have found help children remember their spellings.

We can use different spelling strategies according to a child's preferred style of learning. You have to work out which way he learns best, then tap into it, but it is also important to try to strengthen his weaker or less-used preferences, to make his learning more effective, and create a multisensory experience.

Another tip is to ask your child to spell a word and observe his eye movements to establish learning preference. People move their eyes in certain directions depending on what they are trying to access. Therefore, whether they look up or down, to the left/right, will suggest a particular VAK learning preference. Take a look at the Patterns of Eye Movements table of the different eye cues we use when trying to remember information. Please note: The pictures in the table show what you see when you look at someone who is in the act of remembering. These eye movement patterns typically apply to the majority of *right-handed people*. Left-handed people may show the opposite of these movements.

As with learning any subject, a multisensory approach works best. Instead of just reading or reciting spelling lists, you can sing them, say them to a beat and record them on your computer, iPod or iPhone so you can listen to them as well as read them and make use of diagrams and pictures.

Patterns of Eye Movements

Visual, Auditory and Kinaesthetic

	Facing an individual Remembered image		Facing an individual Constructed image
V Looking up	Visual recalled image (remembered)	Visualising (staring ahead)	Visual constructed (new) image
A Looking towards the ears	Auditory (remembered)		Auditory constructed (new) sound
K Looking down	Internal dialogue (talking to oneself) / auditory		Kinaesthetic / Sensory

VAK/T approaches to spelling

The Visual, Auditory, Kinaesthetic and Tactile (VAK/T) approach uses all the learning preferences. Remember that children with dyslexia often experience 'fuzziness' with auditory and visual senses, so it makes sense to use hands-on, tactile methods, as well as our imagination and a variety of techniques for which your child shows a learning preference.

When learning the way words are spelled (and read), a dyslexic learner needs some tricks to distinguish and remember things like which way the stick goes on a 'b'. Use hand signals and pictures to represent letters.[79] For example, the word 'bed' can be represented as a picture of a bed with the letters 'b' and 'd' forming the bed ends. This helps us remember the orientation of the letters 'b' and 'd'.

How to Remember Which Way Round 'B' and 'D' Go

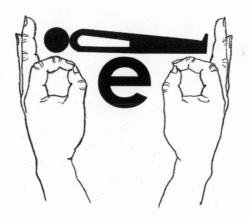

The word bed can also be represented by using your left and right hands to form the letters 'b' and 'd'. If you use the thumb and forefinger to create the circle part, the other three fingers of each hand automatically rise in the correct orientation to complete the letters. The beauty and simplicity of this approach is that a child doesn't even have to remember whether the left or right hand makes the 'b'.

Visual spelling strategies include looking at word shapes, neuro-linguistic programming (NLP) and visualisation, picture associations, pegging, puzzles, word searches and crosswords. You can play board games, card games and create spellings out of pasta, in flour, in sand, with pipe cleaners and even in foam in the bath.

Auditory spelling strategies include listening to the spelling, saying the spelling out loud, songs, rhymes, raps and explanations. Spell the word out loud with large, exaggerated movements of the mouth, while looking at yourself in the mirror. This allows you to 'feel' the way the word is spelled as you pronounce it. If your child is more visual, he may be better with this technique when someone else is saying the word using large movements of the mouth and he is watching, rather than forming, the shapes of the sounds himself.

There are numerous ways to teach kinaesthetic spelling. For example,

- You can make letters out of a tactile material such as soft felt, velvet, dough or clay. Children love to feel and be creative with clay. Make the letters big so that a child can run his hands over them and touch and feel the way words are spelled.

- Using wooden and plastic alphabet letters enables a child to feel the letters in 3D. Letters can be scrambled up and rearranged into order.

- With older children, use stencils that allow you to trace the letter through the stencil. The act of colouring or tracing a stencil allows a child to stare at the letter long enough to begin to lodge it into memory.

- Pebbles appeal to a child's investigative nature. Have fun collecting smooth pebbles. Use permanent coloured markers or paint to write letter sounds on to them. Practise sorting them into sound groups, then mix them up and spell words.

- For a whole-body, kinaesthetic movement, use a piece of carpet and paint lower case letters of the alphabet in squares, so your child can jump from letter to letter and spell out words.

- Use large sweeping movements of the pen when you write the letter. Use recycled paper or invest in flip chart paper, a whiteboard and coloured markers, or a chalkboard and chalks and let your child write huge letters making exaggerated movements.

- Try sky writing (writing in the air) which costs nothing. Children do this with their eyes closed, which is great fun.

The goal of all these techniques is to develop muscle memory and visual memory for letters and groups of letters and then for entire words. Each method provides a new and different texture, feel and experience. Switch them about, keep them the same or use different techniques for different word groups to reinforce the kinaesthetic appeal of different media.

You can try the following tip with words that your child continuously misspells, to develop muscle memory for writing the word correctly. When you write a single word over and over, your brain begins to remember the movements. When we relax and let the brain's autopilot take over, we will begin to write the word correctly over time.

Use coloured pens for words that have similar spelling patterns and similar sounds. Use one colour for one spelling pattern and another colour for a similar sound that has a different spelling pattern. For example:

f-air	f-are	
fl-air	fl-are	
p-air	p-are	p-ear
h-air	h-are	
st-air	st-are	

In this case, column 1 might have red endings, column 2 might be blue, and column 3 green (if your child is colour blind, choose colours he easily recognises – reds and greens are typically difficult to see).

For homophones, words that are spelled differently but have the same pronunciation (e.g. their, there and they're; see and sea; which and witch), I recommend the use of index cards with pictures, mnemonics, colour coding and a short sentence containing the word, to make it memorable.

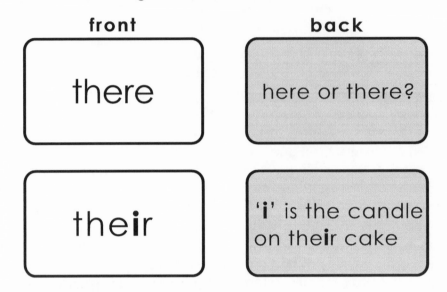

front

there

back

here or there?

their

'**i**' is the candle on the**i**r cake

If your child has an idea of his own for learning to spell, encourage him to try it. After all, he intuitively knows what works best for him. Encourage him also to find his own pictures to represent words because that will help him relate the picture to the word based on his own experience.

When you are helping your child with spelling a particular word, try to expand some of the words into groups with similar spelling patterns or sounds. When you recognise common patterns, point them out to your child and try to reinforce them using the methods described above. Ask your child to think of other words that might have similar spellings (rhyming words) and then explore the spelling of the words your child comes up with and look at why the spelling is or is not the same.

Many students forget how to spell words immediately the spelling test is over. Most non-dyslexic students will eventually relearn some of them with continuous use and regular reading, but a dyslexic student needs more help than learning them once or twice for a test. Try to reinforce spelling over and over, so it is not something quickly learned and quickly forgotten.

NLP Visualisation – Spelling

~ **ou**ght ~

1. Look at the word 'ought'.

   (Take a pretend **photo**)

2. Cover the word with your hand.

3. Form a mental picture.

Now close your eyes. When you are ready, look up left and 'see' the word. (keep repeating steps 1-3 if you need to)

How many letters are there? (= 5)

Are there any v**ow**els? (yes = 2: **ou**)

What **colour** are the vowels? (**ou**ght)

Are there more letters before/after vowel? (0-**ou**-3)

Are there any ta**ll** letters? (yes = 2 oug**ht**)

Are there any descendin**g** letters? (yes = 1 ou**g**ht)

Say the letters in the word out loud? (o-u-g-h-t)

Can you write the word in the air?

Can you write the word in joined-up writing? (*ought*)

Spell it backwards: (t-h-g-u-o)

Spell it forwards: (o-u-g-h-t)

A neuro-linguistic programming (NLP) approach to spelling

In education, NLP is used to improve visual recall of spellings by visualising the word. We look at the shape of a word by identifying letters that are tall or which fall below the line, focusing on the number of vowels and their colours, and the shapes of the consonants (see above for tips on vowel colours). We write the word in the air or with our eyes shut and even read or spell the word backwards! NLP can use all the senses. You can even integrate taste by forming letters cut out of cake or cooked spaghetti and eating them when you have spelled the word correctly.

The table NLP Visualisation - Spelling will help you work through the spelling of 'ought' (there is a mnemonic for this one under Spelling Rules). When your child can spell out a word backwards, he is working hard to visualise the word and, if he can spell it correctly backwards, he will definitely know how to spell it forwards! But even when he gets the spelling of a word correct on several occasions, remember to practise tricky words often so that they are transferred into his long-term memory.

Spelling high-frequency words

Because many high-frequency words do not follow the usual pattern of phonics, most of their spellings cannot be broken down using synthetic phonics. Memorising some of these trickier words can be quite a task for dyslexic learners, so we use flash cards, picture associations and NLP, and the memory strategies we discussed in the **Strategies for successful memorisation**. Using flash cards we write the spelling on the front of the card, and the mnemonic on the reverse.

We even use exaggeration and mispronunciation to spell tricky words. For example, the word 'what' is a high-frequency word and, depending on where you come from, it can have a different correct pronunciation.

In southern England, it is pronounced 'wot'. Sometimes, we purposely mispronounce it 'wat' when trying to learn its spelling. When your child comes to learn how to spell it, you could emphasise 'w-hat' or 'w-h-at' or 'wat with an "h"'. Or remember it's one of the 'wh' question words. Whichever way makes an impact on your child, have fun and laugh at making silly memory links.

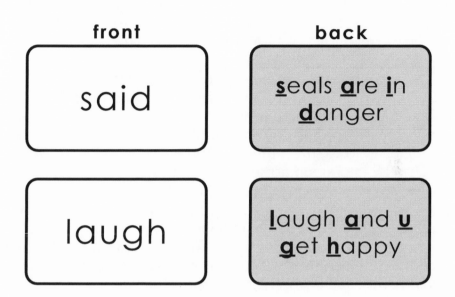

front   **back**

said

seals **a**re **i**n **d**anger

laugh

laugh **a**nd **u** **g**et **h**appy

I have published two multisensory spelling workbooks (I Can Spell – My Spelling Book 1: High Frequency Words and My Spelling Book 2: Medium Frequency Words) that will help your child learn these important high- and medium-frequency words. They employ methods similar to the Look, Write, Cover, Say method used in most schools, but in a much more kinaesthetic and memorable way, including writing with their eyes closed, which children love. It is something parents can help their child with at home.

For tricky spellings, you can make your own flash cards, as above, and have lots of fun with them. Or you can model high-frequency words using clay, Plasticine™, coloured pipe cleaners or any other kinaesthetic method.

The spelling booklets are self-explanatory and easy to use; you can find them at www.icanspell.co.uk.

How to teach English spelling rules and exceptions

Encountering exceptions to spelling rules can be both confusing and frustrating. There is no way around the fact that English is difficult to master. You need a whole separate book for spelling rules and exceptions, so I will give just a taste of a few and how to handle them.

When you encounter words in homework or reading assignments that trip up your child, I recommend dealing with them either one at a time (perhaps as they arise in your child's spelling corrections) or in groups of similar words (depending on your child's ability) in a methodical way. One trick is to draw or print out a picture and paste it on an index card. Write the correct spelling in large letters on the card with the picture, highlight the tricky part, and then simply practise over and over again using a memory technique that suits your child.

Possibly the hardest sound in the English language is the 'gh' sound. Words such as 'though', 'thought', 'laugh' and 'enough' can present challenges. A good way to learn the most common 'gh' words is to tackle most of them in rhyming groups and the rest individually. It helps to separate the 'gh' words from each other, and learn them in rhyming combinations with other word families. For example, some 'gh' words rhyme and are spelled similarly:

- enough
- tough
- rough

However, some sound similar but are spelled completely differently:

- thought
- caught
- sort

Learning spellings in word families with the similar spellings and similar sounds makes remembering much easier. For example:

1. ought

2. **b**ought

3. **br**ought

4. **f**ought

5. **n**ought

6. **s**ought

7. **th**ought

A fun way to remember words ending in 'ought' is to start by making up a mnemonic for 'ought', such as **oh u g**reat **h**airy **t**iger, with a picture of a hairy tiger. Then colour-code the previous one or two letters of the 'ought' word for emphasis and add a picture of someone: 1. With a finger pointing at someone (ought) 2. **B**uying something; 3. **Br**inging something; 4. **F**ighting with someone; 5. Zero; 6. **S**earching for something and 7. **Th**inking about something.

Creating lists of words with similar spelling roots is a good way to learn families of words and their root or stem, such as: **creat**e, **creat**ion, **creat**or and **creat**ive or **famil**y, **famil**iar, **famil**iarity and **famil**iarisation.

We teach readers that the combination of letters t-i-o-n is pronounced 'shun' (position) or 'chun' (question). For words that rhyme with 'ation' or 'otion', or belong to word families, you can create a card with words that follow a pattern, for example:

-motion	-ation
motion	confrontation
emotion	fascination
emotional	hesitation
locomotion	nation
commotion	station

For 'ssion' or 'sion', there is a difference in sound. Words ending in 'ssion', also have the 'shun' sound (as in 'tion'), but in words ending in 'sion', the 's' sounds like a soft 'g' – 'jun':

-ssion	-sion
omission	lesion
commission	decision
permission	television
submission	supervision

Similarly, words like 'bridge', 'edge' and 'hedge' all end in 'dge'. This combination of letters always results in the sound 'j'. You can create a card with words that follow that pattern, too.

When you have identified groups of words as having similar pronunciations and similar spellings, write them together on index cards and refer to them often. I recommend keeping an index card box handy, similar to a recipe index box. Let your child figure out his own scheme for sorting the cards. That way he is more likely to be able to find them. For example, he may choose to sort all words that use a short or long 'o' under 'o' even though the words don't start with the letter 'o'. Words that end in 'tion' might be stored under 't' and words that end in 'sion' might be stored under 's'. Alternatively, post the index cards around the area where he does his homework so he can refer to them without having to search for them, and they serve as a constant reminder.

Don't crowd too many words together on one index card. Between three and five words is more than enough. Use words that your child encounters in reading or subject assignments as much as possible rather than words that are not likely to appear in his everyday vocabulary.

Learning how to write – handwriting

When it comes to helping your child with handwriting, it's important to understand how he controls his fine motor skills. Good posture is important for good handwriting skills. Children should be taught to hold their writing instruments properly using the 'tripod grip'. Small adjustments in holding the pencil can help enormously, as can changing the pencil size or adding a padded pencil grip.

To hold the pencil correctly using the 'tripod grip', the pencil should be positioned so that there is equal pressure between the thumb, the side of the middle finger and the tip of the index finger (the first three fingers including the thumb). All fingers are bent slightly, and the pencil is positioned between all three fingers. A triangular pencil or pen or a pencil grip placed on a standard pencil is particularly useful for positioning the fingers correctly. Nowadays, you can buy pencils and pens designed with indentations to position fingers correctly.

Please do not allow your child to hold his crayon incorrectly. If he picks up a crayon as a toddler in a fist grip, it is going to be much harder for him to hold his pencil correctly later on. I see many children who, at the age of seven, find handwriting tremendously difficult, and the most common reason is that they were not encouraged to persevere with the tripod grip. After the age of six to seven, it is hard for children to undo possibly four or five years of incorrect handwriting technique – so pay special attention to this.

Handwriting - Tripod Grip

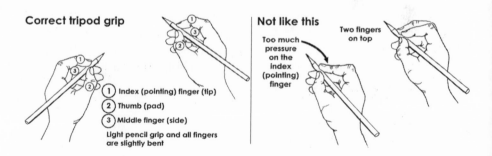

Correct tripod grip

(1) Index (pointing) finger (tip)
(2) Thumb (pad)
(3) Middle finger (side)
Light pencil grip and all fingers are slightly bent

Not like this

Too much pressure on the index (pointing) finger

Two fingers on top

As children write, encourage them to form one letter at a time, paying attention to letter order and the size and spacing of letters and words. Use lined paper to help them write in straight lines. You can use wide-lined paper for younger or less practised children and narrow-lined paper for older or more adept children. When you are happy that all the letters are being formed correctly, you can introduce groups of letters.

Try a tactile approach if your child is having difficulty forming certain letters. Make 3D letters out of play dough or clay. Let your child feel the shape and make them himself. He could then trace over them with his finger and repeat that tracing in sand, using paint, or just on a flat surface. When writing on paper, find a fun pencil, perhaps with a wobbly head on the top, to make the whole experience fun.

I believe children should learn cursive (joined-up) handwriting as early as possible. This involves flowing, almost rhythmic, movements that reinforce patterns and spatial awareness. Most children learn how to print letters first and then move on to cursive handwriting later. Some learners may find it difficult to learn two different types of handwriting so bear this in mind.

The flowing nature of joined-up writing reduces the problems children have with confusing letters or writing 'b' and 'd' backwards. There are theories that suggest that well-formed, flowing handwriting from the outset is linked to spelling ability, as it reinforces left-to-right directionality and spelling patterns.

When exploring handwriting aids, look out for resources that emphasise teaching body and spatial awareness and body posture. If your child is left-handed, look for special help with that since left-handers have to position the pen and paper differently to move across the page fluidly as they write. Other things to check for include your child's visual perception, ocular motor control (using the eyes) and hand-to-eye coordination, and remember to focus on letter orientation and sequencing.

Many schools and teachers have their own handwriting policy, so check to make sure you are both teaching your child the same way. The teacher may even give you a copy of the handwriting programme to practise at home.

Learning how to write stories, essays and reports

Writing stories, essays and reports is notoriously tricky for children who have dyslexia. Putting ideas and words on paper can make them panic. Having a template to fill in makes a massive difference, giving children a much better idea of where and how to start. You can delete the template headings at the end.

Sequencing events is part of the problem. Another problem, due to lack of reading, is that children are not familiar with styles of writing and story plots.

Technology has opened a whole new world to people with dyslexia. It enables them to put ideas down following a sequential layout but, most importantly, technology enables them to move sections around if they are in the wrong order. Even authors use software to help them develop their characters and plot. Technology makes it possible to go back and add fine detail without having to rub text out or scrap it and start again. Progress is seen instantly, which encourages us to write more.

An example of using technology for creative writing is a recent activity I did with 12-year-olds in an extra English progress class. After a term of learning and practising the eight parts of speech (nouns, adjectives, verbs, adverbs, pronouns, prepositions, conjunctions and interjections) and writing sensory descriptions, step by step they pieced their knowledge and ideas together.

The children produced a Venn diagram with pictures of adjectives and descriptions of winter and spring (with an overlap in the middle showing the transition of seasons). First, they typed up their ideas about winter into one paragraph; then they typed up the transition of winter into spring and, finally, they typed up a paragraph about spring. They saved their work and, in subsequent lessons, added more detail. Then, they went back and added exciting openers and conjunctions and then added more adjectives and adverbs. They used the thesaurus facility in Microsoft Word to improve their vocabulary by searching for synonyms of not-so-inspiring adjectives and verbs.

Each lesson, the children were keen to use the computers and were inspired to write without fear. The outcome was stunning – they all produced work that was exciting and inspiring to read. They were so proud of what they had achieved that they all wanted to read out their work.

Younger writers can draw events in a cartoon-style strip, writing a few sentences under each drawing. Later, they can join the sentences together to make a whole paragraph – instant success.

Report writing is much easier using technology. For example, you create main headings and sub headings (using 'styles') and fill in the information underneath. You can even start writing your ideas using bullet points, which makes it easier to piece everything together later into a paragraph. Again, if something is in the wrong order, you can simply select the text and move it, or cut and paste it, into the right location. At the end, you can press the Table of Contents button and, hey presto, you have a contents page.

Teachers receive special training in exactly how to teach reading, spelling and writing to children because it is not easy making sense of the English language and its difficult grammar and spelling rules. Dyslexic learners can learn how to read, spell and write when using multisensory teaching methods and time is taken to teach to their learning preference, strengths and interests. It may take longer, require more patience, and trying out several different methods. There are several remedial literacy programmes available that parents can use at home with their child; recommendations very much depend on what suits your child and what has or has not worked in the past. So you are best seeking advice from a specialist.

Chapter 17
Reading with your child at home

To learn to read is to light a fire; every
syllable that is spelled out is a spark.

Victor Hugo, poet, novelist[80]

Not everybody likes to read. There are still many people in the world who were not taught how to read properly and consequently avoid it at all costs. For others, reading represents the ultimate escape: getting lost in a good novel opens up a world where imagination rules and the impossible happens every day. Regardless of whether or not you enjoy snuggling up in an armchair with a mug of hot tea and good book, it is hard to deny that reading is an essential skill. Children who do not master reading are at a serious disadvantage.

Everyday simple tasks, like filling the car with petrol, withdrawing money at the cash machine, reading labels on food and buying groceries at an automated checkout, all require reading. Interacting with a real person to conduct even the most basic transactions of living is slowly becoming a thing of the past. In today's world, it is increasingly difficult to cope with simple everyday tasks if you cannot read your way through a computerised set of instructions.

If your child cannot read age-appropriate material, he will not only have difficulties in all core subjects at school, but will also suffer from low self-esteem. Reading is a fundamental skill and, if your child can't read curriculum-based material well, he will find tackling maths worded questions very challenging, in spite of being good at mental arithmetic. If he cannot read confidently, he will find reading foreign languages difficult too.

No matter what their inherent talents might be, children who cannot read well and extract meaning from what they are reading are unlikely to perform well in the curriculum and in examinations. Reading is just about the most essential skill a child needs to master. In this chapter, I take apart the process of reading and show you how you can help your child overcome the obstacles that stand between him and the written word.

Why is reading with your child so important?

Educational researchers Herbert Walberg and Shiow-Ling Tsai (1983) found that children entering school with some background in reading and writing are able to get ahead and 'have an abundance' (provided they have been taught correctly), while those who are behind at the starting point seem to lose even more along the way.

In other words, it is important to try to build reading skills early or it becomes harder to catch up later. Special educators can measure a child's reading 'wealth' in terms of letter recognition and phonemic awareness. If a child is having difficulty, early intervention can help a great deal.

In order to build a strong foundation of reading skills, we have to get our children reading and interested in books; children become good readers and writers only by actually reading. Teaching your child how to read will not only improve his academic performance but can be one of the most rewarding experiences you have as a parent. But if your child has dyslexia, it may also be one of the most frustrating and upsetting experiences for you both, if not handled with sensitivity.

> Research shows that parental involvement in their children's learning positively affects the child's academic performance... in both primary and secondary schools... leading to higher academic achievement, greater cognitive competence, greater problem-solving skills, greater school enjoyment, better school attendance and fewer behavioural problems at school.
>
> National Literacy Trust.[81]

If reading is an issue for your child, perhaps causing him high levels of stress and anxiety, you may have reached the stage where you have decided to avoid confrontation and want to leave the reading to the school. Just 20 minutes reading with your child every day will really improve his reading skills. Your input is invaluable and 'more powerful than any other family background variables, such as social class, family size and level of parental education'.[82]

Reading to your child will expose him to a wide range of vocabulary and helps develop important language skills that will help him learn to read on his own. It will help him with creative-writing techniques, effective use of figurative speech, understanding of grammar and syntax, and effective use of punctuation and sequencing skills, all of which are very difficult for a dyslexic learner. It also helps his concentration skills by improving his attention span.

Reading also exposes a child to word structure and sentence building. It is an essential building block in how we learn grammar. As babies, we hear the spoken language around us and assimilate the grammar, but only when we begin to read can we put structure and consistency to grammar and overcome many childish sayings that are the result of mishearing or misunderstanding the spoken language.

There has been much research into the importance of parental involvement in children acquiring literacy skills. The National Literacy Trust website has many free online publications describing research conducted on parental involvement with their child's education.

The following excerpt is taken from *The Importance of Parental Involvement in their Children's Literacy Practices*:

> Involvement with reading activities at home has significant positive influences not only on reading achievement, language comprehension and expressive language skills... but also on pupils' interest in reading, attitudes towards reading and attentiveness in the classroom.[83]

From the time my children were babies, I read to them every night, and they loved it. It was our quiet time together, a time when they had my undivided attention. They would choose a book, searching eagerly through all the pictures first, wondering with excited chatter what the story would be about. Then, all snuggled up, they would wait with anticipation for me to begin reading. They would hang on my every word, taking it all in, predicting what was going to happen next by the tone of my voice. It was exciting for all of us, and we were bonding.

But as they grew older and started to learn how to read, the dynamics of that special experience began to change. As they battled their way through trying to read 'x' number of pages of their school reading book every evening, they became anxious and tense, and our reading sessions became less enjoyable and more of a chore.

My children complained either that they didn't like the story or it was too difficult, too easy or too boring. There were times when even I found some of the stories boring too! Occasionally, the reading level was easy, but the storyline was too childish and, consequently, dull. Their school reading schemes were not inspiring them to read and merely reinforced the fact they found reading really difficult. Sometimes they enjoyed the concept of reading a particular adventure story for their age group, but the book was too difficult for them to decode and, by the time they came to the end of the sentence, they couldn't remember what they had read.

Determined to reinstate the fun in our special reading sessions, I began to search for books that were more inspiring and at their level of reading (and not according to their chronological age). Luckily, I managed to find a wonderful children's book publishing company called Barrington Stoke, which specialises in producing books for reluctant or struggling readers. I recommend publishers and authors at the end of this chapter.

The reading process

We start by learning to read slowly, patiently sounding out every word. We gradually learn to read more fluently. At first, it is easier for us to read out loud, engaging our auditory as well as our visual sense. As we become seasoned and expert readers, we are able to speed up, reading rapidly in our minds, employing some eleven eye muscles to move our eyes from left to right and back again across the printed page. Sometimes we race on, eager to find the point in the material or slow down to decipher a difficult passage. When material is complex, it helps even fluent adult readers to slow down and read a complicated set of instructions or an intellectual hypothesis out loud.

A fluent reader (who is also a fluent thinker) will be able to read a passage and understand it even if words are misspelled or even missing altogether. Fast, intelligent readers may read half sentences, skipping over partial sentences with their eyes and with their brains and predicting the ending faster than their eyes can scan the printed word. This is a way of speed reading.

Despite how it appears to work, the eye cannot actually read while scanning left to right across the page (or right to left for some cultures). Instead, it has to pause for a fraction of a second to focus visually on the written word before moving on. We don't see well when our eyes are moving. We see clearly only when they are still.

When your eye 'fixates' on a word as it is reading, your brain has to decode instantaneously (or as quickly as possible) what it is seeing. Your visual sense passes the information into working memory, where your brain calls on your long-term memory to help decode the word in working memory. Remember that people with dyslexia may have impaired working memory. By the time the long-term memory has decoded the strange set of characters on the page, the working memory may already have forgotten what it saw. No wonder reading is such hard work for people with dyslexia. Be patient with dyslexic readers. They just need longer to focus, to see, to remember and to decode.

One way to help is to use audio along with the written word. When dyslexic readers hear as well as see the writing, it is easier for them to process it. There are many good audio books on the market for all genres and levels of reading, as well as literature books your child will be studying in secondary school.

Unfortunately, much reading has to be done for homework, and reading English literature books can be especially challenging. You have little choice over these books but you can help your child to read them. In general, and apart from assigned homework reading, you can still create a love of reading, even where none exists, by finding the trigger that motivates your child. Perhaps it's reading about their favourite sports team, rock star or actor; or a book about aeroplanes, space exploration or ballet dancing. Every child has a trigger – you just have to find it and then feed it.

In general, stay away from texts that are too difficult, have tiny print or no pictures. Short sentences that are clearly stated in a friendly typeface are best. And PACE yourself. Dyslexic readers need to experience PACE:

**Patience, Awareness, Consistency
and Encouragement**

Tips for choosing books

When you choose books for young dyslexic readers, try using these four steps to check their reading level:

1. Ask your child to open the book at any page

2. Have your child begin reading aloud while you follow alongside him

3. For every mistake he makes, count 1 in your head or on your fingers (make sure he doesn't notice)

4. If, by the end of the page, he has made five mistakes or more, then it is likely that the book is too hard for him.

This 'four-step' approach is by no means scientific, but it's what I use to gauge the reading level of my children. It indicates that, in a given page of the book, a child is encountering too many errors that will probably have an effect on his comprehension. It will also result in frustration and demotivation, which will affect his self-confidence and deter him from reading.

I use the following guideline to gauge the number of mistakes made in a single page of reading:

- If you counted more than five mistakes in one page, the book is too difficult for your child.
- If you counted three to five mistakes, the book should challenge your child and increase his reading skills.
- If you counted fewer than three mistakes, the book should be easy reading and could help him gain fluency.
- It is always best to start with a book that your child can cope with easily, thereby helping him gain confidence.

When selecting a book, look for the following factors:
- Brilliant stories (that you have found, but they have chosen)
- Books and chapters that aren't too long
- Clear and bold fonts, 12–14 point, without italics, preferably printed on off-white or cream-coloured paper
- Short sentences and short paragraphs
- Only left justified i.e. the text is not adjusted to form a straight line on the right-hand side). This helps them identify the sentence length and not lose their place
- For younger children, engaging illustrations that break up the text and help them predict what the text will be about
- For older children, the interest level should be age appropriate.

Children with reading difficulties often experience failure and are consequently not always motivated to read, so the emphasis of reading with your child should be on enjoyment and success. Remember to make it fun and always reward his effort (the Appendix has a reading progress chart).

Set aside a regular slot, when he is not exhausted or hungry, perhaps after supper. All children love positive attention, and knowing that they are going to have your full attention at a certain point in the day will make them feel special, provided it is not fraught with tension! Also, consider the following additional requirements for happy and effective reading times:

- Make sure you have a quiet, comfortable environment
- Read for 20 minutes every day
- Try using a reading ruler or a coloured overlay
- Stop from time to time and talk about the book to check understanding: the plot, the characters and so forth – have fun with it.

When your child struggles to pronounce a word correctly and looks to you for help, break the word down into the separate units of sound (phonemes), blend the sounds of the letters together and break words down into syllables (segmenting). This way you are showing your child the skills needed to decode difficult words. High-frequency 'sight words' will need to be read as 'whole' words.

It is important to emphasise that making mistakes is normal. It is vital not to react by being annoyed or 'shocked', even if he has read the same word correctly many times before or the word seems easy to you.

Shared reading

Shared reading is a technique practised in many schools. Children may be organised into reading groups where each child has to read a couple of sentences out loud. The teacher may supervise the reading or have a parent or helper take part in supervising the group. The same book may be read repeatedly over several days, so that each child will have an opportunity to read a part they haven't read and hear their part read by someone else. The teacher may also stop and talk about the book after each page, or after a significant event takes place in the story.

You can use this technique at home to take the burden out of reading a favourite book. First you read a few sentences, and then your child reads a sentence or two. The next day, you switch and your child reads the part you read and vice versa.

If your child pronounces a word incorrectly or says another word in its place, let him finish the sentence or paragraph before correcting him. He may realise his own mistake, so it is important to give him the chance to self-correct. If you correct every single word he gets wrong, he will feel silly and will become demoralised. Create a safe environment for him to learn and feel good about himself.

Shared Reading with Your Child

The following strategies are valuable when starting to read with your child:

- Ask him to examine the cover illustration and help him read the title.
- Suggest that he predicts what the book might be about, based on the cover illustration, the title, or both.
- Then read the summary at the back of the book and compare it with his prediction.
- Children should make predictions throughout the story and, as they read, and confirm or revise their predictions.
- While reading, always ask questions about the storyline or characters:
- 'What do you think such and such a character is going to do?'
- 'How do you think the character is going to get out of this situation?'
- 'Do you think the character could have done something differently?'
- 'Was that the right thing for the character to have done?'
- 'What do you like about the character or setting, and what would you change?'
- 'Did you expect the book to end this way?' 'How would you have ended it?'

Authors and publishers of dyslexia-friendly books

Barrington Stoke books for reluctant readers

Discovering the Barrington Stoke books for children who find reading difficult completely changed my children's motivation and desire to read. This publisher has a huge selection of fiction genres ranging from exciting adventure stories, ghost stories, comedy and real-life dramas to fascinating facts. Your child will love them. See **www.barringtonstoke.co.uk.** Interest levels are aimed at children between the ages of 8 and 18+. Chapters are short, the font size is slightly larger than normal, and they are printed on off-white paper, making the reading experience for children with dyslexia more pleasurable.

Other valuable resources

Many other publishers and authors have become more dyslexia aware. Waterstones and Dyslexia Action have produced a *Guide to Choosing Dyslexia-Friendly Books for Kids*,[84] listing books by interest level and age group. Some of my personal favourites are:

Jolly Phonics: Uses a multisensory approach with fun characters to teach letter sounds and how they blend to form words. It is also effective for older children who need reading and writing help. **www.jollylearning.co.uk**

The Oxford Reading Tree series by Oxford University Press:[85] Books in this series are designed to teach younger children to read in progressive stages with natural-sounding language. The storylines, characters and illustrations are engaging and provide children with something they can relate to.

The Rapid Reading Series by Heinemann: Has reading intervention programme books and software. Interest level age 7–11+. **www.pearsonschoolsandfecolleges.co.uk.**

Francesca Simon: The Horrid Henry series. Interest level 8–14; reading age 8+.

Roald Dahl: His stories have timeless appeal for children of all ages.

David Orme: The Boffin Boy series has an interest level for ages 8–14; reading age: first series 6–7, second series 7–8.

Andrew McPherson: Retold Text Series is a range of GCSE English literature books. Interest level 14–16+, reading age 8+.

Jacqueline Wilson: This author's website is fun. It has lots of recommendations for children of all ages. **www.jacquelinewilson.co.uk**

Stephanie Baudet: Her books are designed to encourage reading among pupils with a low reading age and high interest age.

David Webb: Has written a wide range of fiction titles for reluctant readers.

Jack Prelutsky: Writes fun poetry books.

For your older reader, Reading Matters is a great website to search for a wide range of topics **www.readingmatters.co.uk**. The Word Pool specialises in books for reluctant readers **www.wordpool.co.uk**.

Downloading books for Kindle or iPad is often cheaper than buying paperbacks, and you can borrow them for free with their lending library service. For children who love technology, using eReaders can create a newfound desire to read that traditional books failed to achieve, possibly because of the connotation of reading being 'hard work'. They can enlarge the print, change background colour and use the built-in dictionary. Several of my students now avidly read books on their Kindle, when previously they had no interest in reading.

All these reading resources make reading as much fun as possible. Try not to get caught up in what a child 'ought to' read. Try to find literature, comics, picture books, annuals, puzzle books, or anything at all that represents the written word, that can help your child nurture a love of reading. A natural curiosity can be explored; a natural gravitation towards a certain topic can be encouraged.

— ✧ —

Chapter 18
Numeracy skills and tips

Do not worry about your problems with
mathematics; I assure you mine are far
greater.

Albert Einstein, physicist, mathematician[86]

Numeracy refers to the ability to manipulate numbers
arithmetically and understand a range of mathematical
concepts. The subject of mathematics is very broad. Beyond the
elementary concept of arithmetic, mathematics includes
geometry, algebra, probability, statistics, trigonometry, calculus
and many more advanced concepts. Because maths is a broad
subject, all the categories may not necessarily be mastered by
one student. Some students may be poor at arithmetic but very
competent in geometry. Others may be good at trigonometry
and calculus, but geometry defeats them.

Around 40-50% of people with dyslexia have no difficulty
with maths. The remaining 50-60% may have difficulties. Some
dyslexic learners may be really good at some of the more
advanced mathematics topics. This is because the dyslexic
brain is particularly good at approaching problem-solving from
multiple angles at once.

Often the challenge is getting children to read and
understand a problem well enough to tackle higher-order
problem-solving. Most tests and exams are written and maths
often includes written problems that requires you to read them,
think them through and work them out on paper in sequenced
steps. Being good at maths can also require a high degree of
self-confidence.

Maths requires strong sequential management. If a dyslexic
learner has a lot of trouble with the concept of time, as many

do, it is likely that this same 'disorientation' will spill over into his sequential reasoning skills. This can present challenges when it comes to higher-order mathematical reasoning of the type required in calculus and higher-level maths.

In general, some difficulties that dyslexic learners may encounter in maths fall into the following categories:

Difficulties in Maths

- Confusion with left/right; clockwise/anti-clockwise
- Difficultly with reading or understanding maths vocabulary
- Difficulty deciding which operations to use to solve problems
- Difficulty decoding word problems
- Difficulty mastering operations such as +, -, x, ÷
- Difficulty remembering and performing sequences in the correct order
- Difficulty reading and interpreting graphs and charts
- Difficulty counting forwards/backwards and counting on
- Impaired concept of time
- Inability automatically to recall facts and figures, such as multiplication tables
- Poor spatial or visual reasoning
- Word or number 'flipping' or transposing.

Writing numbers

Forming numbers correctly is an essential skill and needs to be practised and refined. There is sometimes a dyslexic tendency to write numbers backwards (mirror write) and many children form numbers, incorrectly, from the bottom up. If you notice your child doing this when he is young, spend time trying to correct it early on. It is difficult to break bad habits and incorrect number formation takes longer to rectify as children get older.

The following activities will help your child form numbers correctly:

- Trace over numbers (with arrows to guide)
- Follow dots on paper (with arrows to guide)
- Write numbers using paint, sand or in the air
- Use a blackboard or mini whiteboard
- Use beads or blocks to form numbers
- Say or sing the numbers as you form them

'Reading' mathematics

Just as dyslexic learners sometimes confuse letters, they may also confuse mathematical symbols such as the '+' (add) sign and the 'x' (multiply) sign. They can also inadvertently transpose numbers. While you can guess what they meant when they write 'I went to deb' instead of 'I went to bed,' it is not that easy to guess whether they meant '69' or '96' when solving a mathematical problem.

This problem can be compounded by the fact mathematical phrases such as 'more than' and 'less than' can also confuse dyslexic learners. When asked to evaluate the following phrase, dyslexic learners can experience a great deal of difficulty:

'Is 96 less than or more than 69?'

Often children with dyslexia find it easier to process calculations presented vertically than horizontally. For example, it is easier to process 47 + 26 + 12 = ? written horizontally:

$$TU$$
$$47$$
$$26$$
$$+\underline{12}$$

When working with your child on wordy maths problems, try to break the words and phrases down into simple components (chunks) and work on each component separately. Many children are overwhelmed by the following question even before they have dared to work it out. Seeing a whole pile of words and knowing there are numbers and calculations mixed up in a long sentence causes panic, and they think they cannot do it, so they may not even attempt the question. For example:

Q. Mary is waiting for the school bus that is due to arrive at half past seven in the morning. The journey to school takes thirty minutes. Unfortunately, the bus is running twenty minutes late. What time will Mary arrive at school?

When doing worded maths questions, I ensure that children write the number, any mathematical operation and any other long-hand words **as numbers above the words**. Visually, it makes a big difference to the brain seeing like with like (numbers with numbers).

You can somehow identify patterns better when you are working with similar components. Then children need to work out whether they need to add or subtract 30 minutes and 20 minutes to 7.30 am. (Some children may need help with understanding why and what they need to add or subtract).

Mary is waiting for a bus that is due to arrive at

7.30am
at <u>half past seven</u> in the morning. The journey

+30 min
takes <u>thirty minutes</u>. Unfortunately, the bus is

+20 min
running <u>twenty minutes late</u>. What time will Mary

arrive at school?

Better still, use a timeline and pictures; a visual representation of a maths problem is easier to relate to:

Visual Representation of a Maths Problem

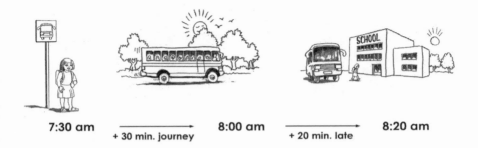

7:30 am $\xrightarrow{\text{+ 30 min. journey}}$ 8:00 am $\xrightarrow{\text{+ 20 min. late}}$ 8:20 am

Basic number skills

Of all the academic subjects, 'reading' maths questions is most likely to cause upset. Keep this in mind and set the stage carefully for maths homework. Make sure your child has as few distractions as possible, keep him engaged in the problems as much as you can, and set incentives and rewards.

If you don't like maths, there are probably more ways you can help your child than you realise. You may think that, because your algebra is rusty or you can't remember Pythagoras's theorem, there is not much you can do, but there are plenty of ways you can encourage and support your child with everyday maths skills.

Making maths fun is the best way to go for young dyslexic learners. And it is easy to have fun with maths by playing board or card games. Another technique is to use a 'chute', where you insert the flash card one way and the answer is on the back. Your child needs to say the answer before the answer comes shooting out at the bottom of the chute.

Using homemade flash cards and other props you have at home, you can play an unlimited number of games to help your child practise the essential basic maths skills listed in the following table.

Basic Maths Skills

- **Review basic mathematical operator language** (add, subtract, multiply and divide) and make sure child understands all the synonyms for the maths symbols:

- **Addition** – add, sum of, plus, altogether, put with, combine, increase, total;

- **Subtraction** – subtract, minus, take away, decrease, less than, fewer than;

- **Multiplication** – lots of, groups of, times, product of, multiplied by, twice/three times, double;

- **Division** – share, divide by, divisible by, half, halve, each, equal groups.

- **Counting** – First, **count all:** 1, 2, 3, 4, 5; then **count on** from a number of items already counted (not starting from 1 again): (5), 6, 7, 8, 9, 10; then **count on from a larger** number (remember the number and do not recount from the beginning to add on more items).

- **Counting backwards** – helps automatic recall. Some children miss out numbers.

- **Number bonds to 10 and 20** – play games and try to learn them by heart! It is best to recall number bonds automatically.

- **Number patterns** – even numbers: 2, 4, 6, 8, 10; odd numbers: 1, 3, 5, 7, 9.

- **Revise and memorise times tables** – using music CDs, games online, your fingers and flash card games such as pairs (see pictures below).

- **Square numbers and square roots** – memorise all square numbers to 10 and square roots to 100 using flash card games such as pairs (see pictures).

- **Estimating** – look at two large numbers and estimate what the sum might be, then add them up and see how close you came.

- **Telling the time** – use an analogue or digital clock (in an ideal world, children need to master analogue time first). Ask questions such as: What time will it be in half an hour? What time was it an hour ago? What time will it be 15 minutes from now?

- **Read a calendar** – look for family birthdays, special days and holidays. Looking at a calendar, ask questions such as: How many days are in the month of July? What day of the week was it on 15 September? What will be the date four Sundays from now?

- **Find some examples of simple graphs** (or make your own) and read the graphs for given values of x and y (x = along the corridor and y = up the stairs). For example, use the x axis for temperature and the y axis for month and plot an approximate curve for the temperature in your local region for different times of the year. Don't worry about being precise – just make an estimate.

- **Make up some maths problems**. Use real objects to make the problem more life-like and fun. Use real apples for this example: Nicky has a basket of apples. If she gives five apples to her best friend Tammy and four apples to her grandmother, and has none left for herself, how many apples did she have in the basket?

When children have automatic recall of basic number facts, they can retrieve answers from memory without having to rely on counting procedures, such as counting on fingers. To help children with memory difficulties, I use props and a·number line to visualise numbers and spot patterns. I use finger games to remember certain times tables, and I let children keep a times tables square in their pencil cases for quick reference – this also helps children become more familiar with the times tables by regularly 'seeing' them. In a non-calculator exam it is very time-consuming to use one's fingers for every calculation – so I teach children how to produce a times tables square quickly and draw a number line at the start of a written exam.

Number bonds

Number bonds are the building blocks of basic addition and subtraction. Children with learning difficulties can find remembering them very tricky. If you make it a top priority to help your child learn them, it will make a great difference to his speed and accuracy of performing mental calculations and spotting number patterns. The key to learning the number bonds is little and often and much repetition and practice.

Repetition, repetition, repetition

You can colour-code the number bonds so that your child can remember that, for example, 3 is yellow and 7 is blue, and draw the corresponding number of objects, so he can count and visualise them (as shown on the flash cards below). You can make up funny number rhymes and songs, or assign objects to different numbers, such as the swan (2) ate two doughnuts (8).

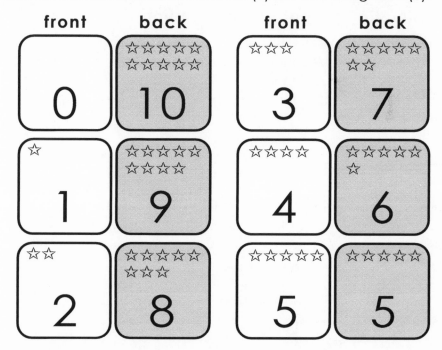

front	back	front	back

Once number bonds to 10 have been mastered using addition, try to learn them using subtraction. A word of warning, children find subtraction much more difficult to master than addition, so you will need to spend much more time on it.

Use real objects to help visualise addition and subtraction concepts. Once your child has mastered both addition and subtraction to and from 10, then show him the relationship between the numbers, as set out in the table.

10 + 0 = 10	10 − 0 = 10
9 + 1 = 10	10 − 1 = 9
8 + 2 = 10	10 − 2 = 8
7 + 3 = 10	10 − 3 = 7
6 + 4 = 10	10 − 4 = 6
5 + 5 = 10	10 − 5 = 5

Eventually, your child can attempt to learn number bonds to 20 in exactly a similar way as to 10. Knowing the bonds will stand him in good stead when identifying more advanced number relationships and number patterns.

Arithmetic and pattern recognition

The ability to be good at maths can depend in part on our ability for pattern recognition. Think of our numbering system (1–10, 10–100, 100–1000 and so on). Think of the enormous number of patterns in maths. Here are a couple more that most of us are familiar with:

$$3 + 7 = 10$$
$$30 + 70 = 100$$
$$300 + 700 = 1000$$

Take a look at the pattern of the nine times tables:

1 x 9 = 9	(0+9 = 9)
2 x 9 = 18	(1+8 = 9)
3 x 9 = 27	(2+7 = 9)
4 x 9 = 36	(3+6 = 9)
5 x 9 = 45	(4+5 = 9)
6 x 9 = 54	(5+4 = 9)
7 x 9 = 63	(6+3 = 9)
8 x 9 = 72	(7+2 = 9)
9 x 9 = 81	(8+1 = 9)
10 x 9 = 90	(9+0 = 9)

There are countless other patterns of increasing complexity in arithmetic. Some dyslexic learners have trouble with sequencing, which can make it harder to recognise patterns. With your help (or the help of his teacher) he can focus on the basic concepts of arithmetic.

Start with basic counting up to 100 and backwards from 100 to 1 and then move on to simple arithmetic concepts of addition, subtraction, multiplication and division. Work with small numbers until he grasps the concept and then try extending the concept to harder numbers. Counting *6 backwards and forwards (even just from 1 to 10) is good practice at sequencing for a dyslexic student.

Point out areas when sequencing is not a problem. For example, 25 + 46 results in the exact same answer as 46 + 25. However 46 – 25 (= 21) will have a different answer from 25 – 46 (which equals -21, a negative number).

Sequencing and pattern recognition also come into play when trying to make sense of formulae. Additionally, the reasoning behind formulae can be perplexing. In the same way that some people with dyslexia can read a book from cover to cover and still not grasp the big picture plot, they can study many components of a formula or even derive a formula for themselves and still not see the purpose of its application or be able to solve a problem that requires its use.

Remember that some of a dyslexic learner's problems are not an inherent lack of understanding of the concept of arithmetic, but rather the more practical issues of identifying patterns, reading word problems, short-term memory or speed of processing.

Times tables and multiplication facts

The times tables are the foundation of your child's numeracy education. It is an important skill to be able to multiply not just at school, but at home, work and play. For dyslexic learners, the times tables are among the most challenging areas in terms of being able to remember and recall number facts. The most effective way of making them more memorable is by using fun rhymes and musical CDs to help children make connections and links.

Did you know that your child needs to grasp only 36 facts to know all the times tables up to 10? Once your child has learned the 2s, 5s and 10s (in and out of order), teach them: 3x3; 4x4; 6x6; 7x7; 8x8; 9x9 by heart too. These are not only important to know by heart for learning square numbers and square roots, but they also serve as an effective strategy to help children obtain the remaining facts by adding on or taking away from these numbers if they are unable to commit all the tables to memory.

One way to help children make progress is to break the tables up into small manageable chunks, showing them how to achieve one thing at a time. We do this by learning a few of one set of tables at a time, then going back and making sure that they still remember the previous set learned. It is vital to show children how much they already know since that can go a long way towards encouraging them to keep on trying. They need to continue to revise the ones they have already learned before learning a new set. Remember to teach them that 6x7 is the same as 7x6.

Children need to practise them over and over again before they become automatic. There are many tips and tricks to learning the tables, but the most important consideration is to make it fun by incorporating sing-song rhythms, dance, arm movements and funny rhymes.

Learning multiplication facts or the times tables can be demoralising for your child, particularly if he finds it difficult to remember. Rather than have an endless battle trying to learn them by reciting them aloud, you can use games with counters or sweets, interactive computer games, apps or musical methods, which also make them much more memorable. My pupils love using their hands and fingers to remember the 9 times tables. You can also use your fingers for the 3 times and 6 times too by counting the natural creases in your fingers.

A good prop for the times tables is to make a chart with the numbers 1 to 12 along the top and along the left-hand side and fill in all the values in the cells in between. Let your child slide his fingers along the top and down the left side to locate the correct answer in the grid. You can make a small grid that can be kept in a pencil case for easy reference or a large grid to put on a wall for easy visual reference at any time. Let your child colour the number patterns in the grid or place coloured bingo counters on the same numbers everywhere they appear in the grid and explore the patterns the bingo counters make. Now rearrange the counters to find numbers that ascend and descend by two, three, etc. Your child is best trying to learn square roots and square numbers by heart (diagonally highlighted on the Times Table Chart).

Times Tables Chart

1	2	3	4	5	6	7	8	9	10
2	4	6	8	10	12	14	16	18	20
3	6	9	12	15	18	21	24	27	30
4	8	12	16	20	24	28	32	36	40
5	10	15	20	25	30	35	40	45	50
6	12	18	24	30	36	42	48	54	60
7	14	21	28	35	42	49	56	63	70
8	16	24	32	40	48	56	64	72	80
9	18	27	36	45	54	63	72	81	90
10	20	30	40	50	60	70	80	90	100

As many children find it too difficult to learn their tables automatically and out of order, a good strategy is for your child to produce his own tables square and to practise doing this at speed. If he spends five minutes at the beginning of a maths exam writing out the times tables square, it will give him the confidence and speed to answer questions accurately throughout the exam. You can download free empty times tables grids and partially completed grids from many websites, so that your child can practise completing them.

How to Remember the 9 Times Tables

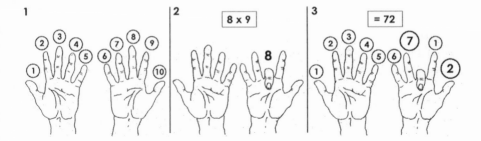

Hold your hands up with your palms facing you. Number your fingers from left to right as 1 to 10.

Now hold down the finger of the number you want to multiply by 9, e.g. to multiply by 8 (8 x 9), bend your 8th finger.

Your fingers to the left are the 10s and the fingers to the right are the units, i.e. there are 7 fingers to the left of your bent finger and 2 to the right, which makes 72.

Making flash cards and playing games

Flash cards are also great for learning the times tables and improving memory skills: E.g. write '4 x 6' on one flash card and write the answer '24' on a different-coloured card to easily identify question and answer cards. Place all cards face down on the table. As your child picks up a sum card, he says 4 x 6 equals 24, and picks up a card of the other colour to find the answer. Each time, he will also use his memory skills to remember where the cards are located. Or write the question on the front and the answer on the back and use a chute for cards.

Money

Children love handling money and counting money out, but find calculating change quite tricky. Making your child responsible for money early on is a good way to teach him how to manage and be responsible about money and to save up for things he really wants to buy.

Play shops when they are very young. Use plastic or real money and practise different ways to give change. Or draw some coins on pieces of paper and cut them out for an unlimited supply – but I can guarantee you the real thing will keep your child's interest much longer. Get your older child to be responsible for paying for the shopping when you are out together.

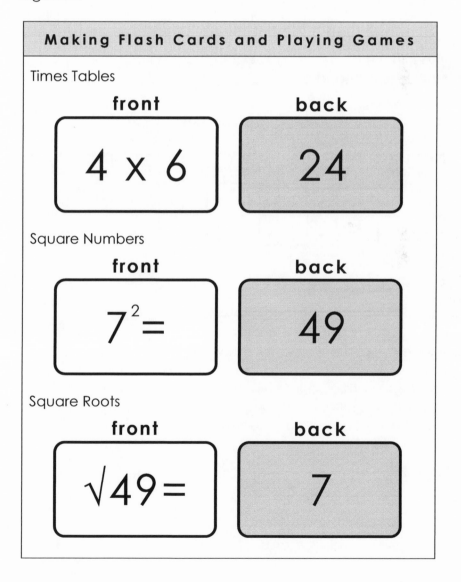

Making Flash Cards and Playing Games

Times Tables

front

$$4 \times 6$$

back

$$24$$

Square Numbers

front

$$7^2=$$

back

$$49$$

Square Roots

front

$$\sqrt{49}=$$

back

$$7$$

Fractions and decimals

Once your child has mastered the basics, begin to work with more complex concepts such as fractions and decimals. Use the multisensory techniques such as plastic fraction parts or a pizza to show individual fractions and fractions that are similar (e.g. 2/4 is the same as 1/2 – then write it down 2/4 = 1/2; 3/6 = 1/2; 4/8 = 1/2; 5/10 = 1/2). Remember to practise regularly and be patient. Your child will remember one day and forget the next if you do not practise frequently – little and often.

Set out decimals using a place value grid. Many children find the concept quite challenging. Ask them to write the number in the grid, so they are able to read it more easily: twenty five thousand and sixty four point one nine (25,064.19)

Place Value Chart

Million			,	Thousand			,	H	T	U	•	Tenth	Hundredth
h	t	u	,	h	t	u	,	h	t	u	•	1/10	1/100
			,		2	5	,	0	6	4	•	1	9

Cooking by numbers

Kids love cooking, especially with a friend or adult! Adolescents enjoy it too. Children are never too old to get pleasure out of rolling up their sleeves and getting stuck in. They love the undivided attention, being creative and, the best bit of all: the reward of munching through what they have created with you or their friends. Helping them to prepare their favourite meal or baking cakes is an ideal way to get them familiar and comfortable with maths such as:

- reading and interpreting new language
- concept of measuring
- concept of weighing
- grams and kilograms

- millilitres and litres
- solids versus liquids
- doubling (ingredients)
- calculating cooking time
- doing things in sequence
- ratios (1 egg to 100g of flour)
- temperature (Celsius versus Fahrenheit)
- fractions (serving up portions or parts of a whole cake)
- number skills: setting the table for six people

There is no doubt that cooking improves maths skills, is pleasurable and unites a family through social interaction.

Gardening by maths

Young children in particular enjoy being and working with you in the garden – if you can get your older child to help you in the garden, then I take my hat off to you! Gardening creates many opportunities to learn more about maths through play and interaction, such as:

- patterns and shapes: of plants, paving slabs, walls
- length: short/tall; more than, less than, the difference between
- counting: bulbs in 1s, 2s, 3s, 4s and 5s
- measuring: spacing out bulbs evenly every 20 cm
- measuring liquid: giving 100ml to each new seedling
- temperature: greenhouse versus outdoors
- ordering: pot sizes, position of plants
- categorising: objects or insects
- area: amount of manure needed
- perimeter: of fencing, lawn
- geometry and symmetry: plants, insects
- even trigonometry and algebra!

The maths opportunities are endless in the outdoors; it doesn't feel like formal learning and children are less likely to get stressed out. It is fun, kinaesthetic learning that is well suited to dyslexic learners.

Games and technical props

Playing games with your child can help with mathematical facts and arithmetic rules just as it can with learning to read and to spell. Use a deck of cards to play Blackjack for example, or make up your own game, such as arithmetic poker. Count the picture cards as 10 and the aces as 11 and then deal out five cards. The person whose cards total the most is the winner. Use poker rules to determine whether you want to allow drawing from the deck a certain number of times. Give your child plenty of time to add the numbers and provide a calculator for a quick check rather than let him become discouraged.

Bingo is a good game to become familiar with recognising basic numbers in the right order and also helps to develop pattern-recognition skills. Games that use one or two dice are also helpful even if the game itself is not necessarily about numbers. Play a game of Monopoly® or try a game of poker dice, which uses up to five dice, to up the stakes.

Let your child use a calculator. Use a handheld one or a giant coloured one, the one on your computer or even the one on your mobile phone. Do whatever makes the learning fun and easy.

Another great tool for older learners who enjoy using computers is learning how to use a spreadsheet. Excel is a powerful calculating tool capable of handling multiple equations and formulae. Use it to check arithmetic, learn the basics of equations and so on. There are free spreadsheet apps you can download on iPad and iPhone too.

Maths and cognitive development

For children who do not have dyslexia, it can be enough to learn that when you see an addition sign you add the numbers on the left and right of the sign together. For dyslexic learners, the process for solving maths problems is more easily mastered when it is connected to a conceptual idea. Using real items and props helps dyslexic learners to develop intangible concepts into more meaningful ones and the hands-on experience sinks more deeply into the memory. If you have insufficient props available, improvise or draw pictures.

As with other types of learning, mathematics should be taught at a level that is appropriate to a child's cognitive development. If you try to teach concepts that are beyond the maturity of a child's thinking, then your approach is doomed to failure no matter how bright the child and no matter whether or not he has dyslexia. It will be difficult, if not impossible, to teach abstract mathematical concepts to a child who has not reached the abstract level of cognitive development (which begins around age ten or twelve and may not fully develop until the later secondary or high school years).

Similarly, if specific difficulties inherent in dyslexia (such as poor short-term memory and difficulty processing multiple instructions) make it hard for a child to listen to instructions and remember what is being said, explore new approaches to teaching and learning. This will involve breaking the problem down into smaller, more manageable problems, and into small, easy-to-understand steps. Write the steps down on an index card for your child to refer to again and again, and save them for when he has to revise for a maths test later in the term.

Maths is traditionally a problem area for many students. Among both girls and boys, it may be a leading cause of upset and feelings of low self-esteem at school. If your older child is sitting important exams, and just cannot understand certain maths concepts, give him a boost by asking for help from a teacher, friend, older sibling or getting a tutor if you can afford it. I strongly recommend it, as most further education requires having passes in both maths and English.

Chapter 19
Art and music

Neither a lofty degree of intelligence nor imagination nor both together go to the making of genius. Love, love, love, that is the soul of genius.

*Wolfgang Amadeus Mozart,
composer, musicia*[87]

Art has long been used by psychologists as a means to understand what children are thinking. A picture that makes use of heavily scribbled black lines going around in circles conveys a very different mood from a picture of a cottage, a sun, and a stick person with a smiling face.

As well as being therapeutic as a means of self-expression, doodling, colouring and sketching are great ways to keep an active child occupied and out of trouble. For those who enjoy it, art is also a great way to relax and relieve stress.

Arts and crafts are kinaesthetic subjects. You can move freely around an art table, wander off to get supplies or replenish your painting water. For children who have trouble sitting still, it can be a relief to be able to get up and move around as they work.

A wide range of different materials and media can be employed in artistic creations. Modelling with Plasticine™, painting with watercolours, sketching with pastels and making things from craft paper are excellent ways to channel artistic talents. But don't stop there. Explore beading, sculpting, pottery and a whole host of other artistic endeavours.

When a child looks upon his own artistic creation, it is generally with a sense of pride. The picture doesn't have to be that great; just the act of creating it is satisfying. Art is good for the soul and allows children to explore their personality and express themselves. It is not important whether a child is talented at art in order for him to find expression and relaxation in it. A child who finds drawing frustrating might enjoy a paint-by-numbers set or a colouring book and set of coloured pencils. Children can also gain great enjoyment from looking at art. They can appreciate colour and texture, shapes and themes. As they grow older, they may also appreciate symbolism in art and show preferences for one style over another. Awakening an appreciation of art in your child can lead to a greater tendency towards creative problem-solving. It also helps to develop fine motor skills, which can be a big help if your child has a tendency towards dyspraxia.

Educators have long believed there is a connection between art and other skills such as maths and languages. In 2005, the University of Colorado at Boulder ran a project and conference to study the connection between maths and art.[88] Carla Farsi, who led the study, claims that, since mathematics is based on the science of pattern and structure, it resembles art, which is similarly based on patterns and structure. The conference explored themes such as computer-generated art, which is a combination of mathematical algorithms and artistic talent – 3-D visualisation and computer-aided modelling programmes rely heavily on both. Artistic handicrafts such as quilting and knitting rely heavily on mathematical calculations, symmetry and geometry.

There are many ways to channel the artistic talents of a child with dyslexia in the classroom. For example, we can encourage children to use a variety of coloured pens to draw images and lines and create a visual Mind Map® for an essay outline or attention-grabbing posters. They can create graffiti boards to become emotionally engaged and to brainstorm ideas for writing assignments or revising.

A child who doesn't enjoy drawing may love poetry, which is also a form of artistic expression. Using computer software to write poetry or song lyrics can alleviate much of the stress of writing assignments or remembering spellings, and yet allows a child the freedom of self-expression.

Art therapy

Art therapy gives children and adolescents, especially those with learning disabilities, a way to build self-esteem and confidence. It is a holistic programme that uses the creative process of art-making as well as therapeutic counselling to improve and enhance the physical, mental and emotional well-being of children, adolescents and adults of all ages. It is based on the belief that the creative process involved in artistic self-expression helps children manage behaviour, reduce stress, increase self-esteem and self-awareness, develop interpersonal skills and resolve inner conflicts.

Art therapy can help children with emotional and behavioural difficulties, speech and language problems or any stress-related problem. It helps a child release bottled-up emotions such as frustration, anger or sadness, through freedom of expression and expert therapy sessions. It gives children a way to express themselves through interpretation and nonverbal communication.

Through the making of images and models, and by the act of 'playing' with art materials, a child is able to express some of his inner world of thoughts and feelings. For example, continually smoothing the surface of a piece of clay with a sponge may achieve a calming effect. The act of creating art is used as a basis for discussion of emotions and also leads to increased self-confidence and self-accomplishment.

The following is a list of some art therapy organisations across the world where you can find out more information:

- British Association of Art Therapists
- American Art Therapy Association
- International Expressive Arts Therapy (US)
- Arts in Therapy (US)
- Canadian Art Therapy Association
- ANZATA (Australia and New Zealand)
- Australian Creative Arts Therapy Association
- Art Therapy India
- Lefika La Phodiso – The Art Therapy Centre (S. Africa).

Music

Music is art you can hear. Listening to music is one of the most popular ways to relax. A good beat is useful when you are working out, walking the dog or doing housework. Many students, including children, can focus better on their homework with music lightly playing in the background. Musical notes resonate in the human body and stir vibrations. Certain notes can create specific moods in people, hence the expression 'mood music'. There is music that helps you focus, music that gets you going and music that lifts your spirit when you are down.

Playing music can have a similar effect as listening to it, with the added benefit that actively participating in the creation of music can give vent to self-expression in the same way as art can. If you compose and play your own music, this becomes even more true, but even playing another composer's music can give you a feeling of power, control and self-expression. It is good for the soul, engages the mind and boosts self-esteem.

Moira Thomson,[89] writing for Dyslexia Scotland, notes that music helps learning in other subjects too:

> Success in musical activity can boost a dyslexic pupil's self-esteem and can encourage re-visiting of other learning areas which might have seemed difficult previously.

For some time now, scientists have been telling us that playing a musical instrument can help children learn better in school. Numerous studies have been conducted that conclude that music helps people learn better and enhances cognitive development.[90] Dr James Catterall of UCLA[91] led a ten-year study to look at the effects of art and neuroscience. He concluded that students involved in music achieve higher marks in standardised tests. There is evidence that music helps to sharpen hearing and sharpen the brain.[92] Look at the research papers at **www.musicandthebrain.org** on the science behind learning and music for further in-depth reading.

Tuning in to musical notes and vibrations can also help us tune in to other sounds, such as speech or the tone of someone's voice, and make us better at listening. The brain trained early in music develops an acute auditory sense and improves memory and attention span. Gottfried Schlaug, in a study conducted at Harvard University,[93] determined that early music training improves motor and auditory skills as well as verbal and non-verbal reasoning. This connection was found to be particularly striking in young dyslexic learners, suggesting that musical education is especially beneficial for people with dyslexia. The ages of 10 to 13 proved especially susceptible to mind strengthening in concert with musical training.

Music is also helpful for reading skills. Using rhythm and sounds can help children remember written or printed words. If your child is motivated by rhythm, sounds and song, take a look at the Thrass approach,[94] which uses music to teach reading. Encourage older children to find the lyrics to their favourite rock songs either in a CD jacket or by searching on the Internet. Many song lyrics are freely available.

Rhymes and rhythm are well-used and well-proven techniques to help dyslexic learners remember things. You can set almost anything to music or to the beat of a drum. Turn a boring set of history dates or a mathematical formula into a rap song or say it over to the rhythmic beat of a bongo drum.

Music and dyslexia

As with all other subjects, your child may or may not experience a variety of symptoms associated with his dyslexia while learning music. For example, he may have trouble with understanding or remembering the musical notation. This may in part be caused by difficulty with processing the music visually and poor short-term memory, making it hard for him to listen while it is being explained. He may also experience difficulty with the fingering and manual dexterity required by nearly all musical instruments. The reverse of this is also true – he may have above normal competence at fingering and playing.

Some dyslexic students may be naturally gifted at playing music but have trouble reading it. These children may need additional support and encouragement to learn to read the notes. Improvisation is a wonderful skill but true musical ability requires a combination of skills, including improvisation, memorisation and sight reading.

Other side-effects of dyslexia may include blurring or fuzziness when looking at the black and white notes. One trick to overcome this is to use coloured overlays. This helps distinguish different notes as well as reduce the glare that comes from the stark contrast between black and white.

Another helpful trick is to rewrite complex passages of music where notes are extremely crowded together into more widely-spaced passages to make them easier to read. With beginners, you can skip musical notation altogether and simply write the letter names of familiar tunes on a piece of paper, while teaching children the correct rhythm and beat for the music. You can gradually introduce musical notation once a confidence in playing and a love of the instrument are established.

Other symptoms of dyslexia, such as forgetting to bring music to the music lesson, forgetting to practise, and general disorganisation, are no less at play in this area than in other areas of your child's life. Don't automatically interpret these general signs of dyslexia as a lack of interest in music.

If the interest in playing a musical instrument is there, you (or the music teacher) may have to work very hard at helping him acquire automaticity (the ability to master something through constant practice).

Working on problem areas in music is much like working on problem areas in other subjects. Use multisensory learning techniques and plenty of repetition, which is vital to developing the kind of automaticity required for playing an instrument. Skill at playing depends in large part on a combination of manual dexterity coupled with rote memorisation. Frequent practice ensures that muscle memory is developed for playing complicated musical passages, scales and so on. Remember, it is easier for children with dyslexia to learn when material is broken up into small chunks. Learning a few lines of music at a time is quite enough. There is no need to tackle a whole piece in a single lesson.

Since dyslexic learners sometimes have trouble with sequencing the 'whole picture', it can be useful if a teacher or another student plays the piece all the way through before it is broken down into chunks for learning. This gives the student an overall way ahead and a good feel for the music. Sometimes, it is also useful to hear it played by a professional orchestra, perhaps on a CD recording, but this can also be overwhelming for someone new to an instrument and who cannot play fast or particularly well.

Many children with dyslexia are very good at playing the piano but, while they are learning, remember this calls on skills not required by other musical instruments, such as reading two lines of music at once for the left and right hands. The musical staves are different, meaning the notes for the left-hand (bass clef) are in different positions on the musical stave from the notes for the right hand (treble clef). This means learning two sets of musical notations, not just one. Add to that the difficulty of having to coordinate two hands playing different sets of notes at the same time, and it becomes quite challenging.

Mastering the piano is an excellent foundation for building concentration and focus in the brain, as well as manual dexterity. It is also a good counterbalance for wrists and fingers that might spend too much time at the computer. So I strongly encourage patience and perseverance with the instrument if your child shows any interest.

Music therapy

If your child suffers from stress, behavioural or emotional difficulties due to a learning difficulty or other personal circumstances, music therapy may help improve his emotional well-being. Music therapy is a therapeutic non-verbal programme that uses music and therapy as a means of reaching non-musical goals.

There are hundreds of research articles in the British Journal of Music Therapy that suggest there are parallels between rhythm and motor behaviour; speech and expressing oneself and singing; and musical mnemonics and rote memorisation. Music therapy is also designed to enhance mood, attention and behaviour and improve the ability to learn and interact.

Children do not need musical training to benefit from music therapy, but it is often the case that children with learning difficulties enjoy music. So it could be that your child enjoys using music as a medium to express his feelings. The process is designed to help children express themselves better, become more aware of their feelings, manage stress and communicate more easily.

It is also used to help people with auditory difficulties, dyslexia, ADHD, autism and other learning difficulties by helping improve the auditory discrimination of sounds; and it can enhance memory, improve organisational skills and alleviate pain.

Music therapists are professionals who have trained for many years in music and psychology and helping individuals with learning disabilities, physical, emotional and psychological disorders and sensory impairments. Music therapists work with children, adolescents and adults of all ages, even pre-school children. Involving a child in creative music-making can also help his physical awareness and develop attention, memory and concentration skills.

The following is a list of some of the music therapy organisations across the world where you can find out more information online:

- British Society for Music Therapy
- American Music Therapy Association
- Music Therapy World (European Music Therapy Confederation)
- Australian Music Therapy Association
- Nordoff-Robbins (Worldwide)
- Association for Professional Music Therapists (UK)

The Mozart Effect®

Don Campbell is a professional music critic and teacher who has travelled the world using music as therapy. He has spent many years studying the healing effects of music on a variety of conditions, and has written several books about what he terms 'The Mozart Effect®'.[95]

This refers to the 'transformational powers of music in health, education and well-being'. Mr Campbell has effectively used music to relieve symptoms of stress and anxiety, improve the ability to relax and improve memory and awareness. He claims that his techniques also work to improve symptoms of dyslexia, ADD and ADHD, and autism, among others. The technique is based on Mozart's music, especially his violin concertos and symphonies, which contain passages of high-frequency sound.

Campbell has found that the high-frequency sounds produced in a beautiful and compelling way by Mozart's superb talent stimulate the auditory system. He compiles various albums combining slow, soothing music at lower frequencies designed for relaxation with high-frequency music to stimulate learning and attentiveness. The healing power of music is related to its ability to vibrate within the body, provoking emotions and creating feelings of harmony or disharmony, depending on the music. To learn more about the Mozart Effect®, visit Don Campbell's website at **www.mozarteffect.com**.

Music and art classes

Being talented at art and music is usually recognisable quite early in children. A five-year-old may demonstrate interest in an old musical instrument lying around the house or may beg for a toy piano, saxophone or guitar. It might be worth enrolling a child who shows interest in music in a music class. If his interest grows, music can be a wonderful outlet that can last a lifetime as a hobby or grow into something more.

If you think music lessons would be a good idea for your child, start early if possible. As a child grows older, it is harder, not necessarily to learn a musical instrument, but to find the interest to begin and sustain the practice. Catching the talent early locks it in and helps the child establish a love for it. If practising an instrument is a chore you have to nag your child into, maybe music lessons are not the right way to go. If it's not fun, it will not have the therapeutic value of a beloved hobby.

When looking for a music teacher, ask if the teacher has any experience with dyslexia. You also want to ensure that the teacher has the experience working with children who have difficulty in reading musical notes, short-term memory or speed of processing problems for example. Look for a general awareness of the special teaching needs required by dyslexic students – or at least a willingness to work with you and your child in a helpful way.

Take a look into the Suzuki approach,[96] a holistic approach to music teaching that is beneficial for dyslexic learners. The Royal School of Music will make special provisions, for example, if made aware of a student's dyslexia, such as extra time for examinations, especially sight-reading, as well as special seating or lighting arrangements. It may also allow students to bring their own music that has been adapted with colours and special markings.

Many communities offer a variety of art classes, pottery, crafts or design classes for children at art schools, exhibition centres and fine arts associations.

Encouraging art and music at home

Here are some fun ways to nurture a love for the arts and music in your child:

- **Play an instrument in the home**. If you play an instrument yourself, play it sometimes when your children are in earshot. Even though they may be playing their own games, they will absorb the atmosphere of the music and learn to love it.

- **Play music at home**. Build a library of different types of music (e.g. guitar solos, light classical music, rhythmic music, world music, opera and music written especially for children).

- **Try out toy instruments** such as tambourines, drums, piano and guitar and see what he gravitates towards.

- **Rent an instrument** before agreeing to buy one. This gives your child time to try out different instruments before you invest heavily in something that might be abandoned after a few months.

- **Do family art projects together**. Putting together a scrapbook is a great way to start, collecting photos for a family album or making cookbooks from your favourite family recipes.

- **Create a special art cupboard** or drawer for art supplies so that all the things you need are in one place and your child knows where to find them. Include paste, glue sticks, colouring pencils, water colours, paintbrushes and sponges, craft paper, plain white paper and so on.

- **Go on outings** to local schools, colleges, the library and civic theatres to see plays, musical performances or art exhibitions. Talk about the costumes, the music, the scene changes and the different art media

- **Expose your child to a variety of art topics** by getting books from the library and looking for good DVD or TV documentaries on topics such as glass-blowing, sculpture, jewellery design, car design, fashion design, interior decorating.

The arts and music are wonderful outlets for being creative, releasing emotion and relaxing. Similar benefits can also be derived from doing physical activity and sport. Such activities not only provide children with pleasure and emotional well-being, they can help with energy levels at school, helping children cope better with the stresses of academic demands.

Chapter 20
Sport and Exercise

If I wasn't dyslexic, I probably wouldn't have
won the Games. If I had been a better
reader, then that would have come easily,
sports would have come easily... and I never
would have realised that the way you get
ahead in life is hard work.

Bruce Jenner, Olympic athlete[97]

B eing involved with a sports programme or physical activity is
usually extremely beneficial for all children. If sport did
nothing other than boost self-confidence, I would recommend
it for that reason alone. Children with dyslexia especially benefit
from participating in sports. Many dyslexic learners whom I
coach are naturally very talented at sports; others have
developed an interest that has become a passion.

Being good at something and having the chance to prove
it often is very good for your spirit and emotional well-being.
Practising sports keeps you physically fit, improves blood
circulation and boosts your immune system. People who are
physically active catch fewer colds, fight them off more quickly
and otherwise have a greater tendency to fight off infections.

Participating in a sports team is a great way to improve
your natural athletic ability and to have fun and make
friendships. Sports teams can be very tight knit and children can
develop lifelong friendships with team members.

Children who enjoy playing sports gain respect for
themselves and for others. They are less likely to suffer abuse
from other children because athletic ability is generally
respected by secondary-aged school students as being hero-

like. What's more, many schools attach great importance to their sporting players and give them high visibility in school. If their games or events are attended by other students from the school, there is nothing like being cheered on by your peers as you make a winning pass, score a goal or hand off successfully to another player from across the pitch. For dyslexic learners who may feel humiliation in the classroom, being cheered on by peers outside class gives a whole new dimension to experiencing self-respect.

Improved coordination through sports can lead to improved coordination in other things. Core strength improves balance; balance improves core strength. (Balance and core strength develop naturally as a result of activities such as martial arts, yoga, tai chi and Pilates.) Improved reaction and response times will help as teenagers prepare for activities such as driving.

Working with a team helps to improve interpersonal skills in general, which will spill over into all aspects of a child's life even as he grows into adulthood. Sports also make you mentally tough; you learn to handle failure and to persevere. You also learn to play by the rules and that the rules matter. Children need to let off steam, and sports can provide a valuable social arena, often the only one, for interacting with peers, but it can provide children with good opportunities to develop friendships, camaraderie, a healthy mind and a healthy body.

For children, who suffer from poor body image, sports can improve feelings of self-worth and greatly improve body image. Girls who play sports are apparently less likely to become pregnant while still at school, less likely to smoke, and more likely to complete their secondary education.

An organised athletic activity can provide positive interaction with adults. Team coaches are authority figures and positive role models who are generally respected team members. A coach shapes a student's commitment to the sport but also grows to respect and admire that commitment over time. For dyslexic students who may experience poor interaction with teachers of academic subjects who do not completely understand why they are not performing in the classroom, having other (non-family) adult role models who praise and encourage them can be a much-needed breath of fresh air. A team sport involves hard work and commitment and coaches and team members often get to know each other quite well.

It is a matter of personality and personal preference whether your child chooses to engage in an activity that is a team effort, such as football or basketball, or something that is an individual sport, like taekwondo or karate. Both have advantages and disadvantages, and offer competition-level participation. You might also look into one-on-one sports, such as tennis or squash, that foster individual competition but can be team sports (doubles) and can also be played with regular special friends. This might work for someone who is quiet or shy, but who still wants to do sport with a trusted friend or family member to develop athletic ability.

Pressure from over-commitment

If you have a young athlete superstar on your hands, your child may have difficulty choosing between different sports, and may have committed himself to many activities. You may find yourself flying around to several events after school, which won't help him in the long term. Sports can be an intense commitment physically and in terms of the time required. Over-commitment can affect the quality of and attitude to homework, and in some cases, lead to falling behind with school work. The aim is to strike a good balance between school work and out of school activities.

Excellence is satisfying

When children become good at something, the feeling of achievement ripples over into other aspects of their lives. Often just one pick-me-up can cure a whole host of issues. It can help children realise a sense of control over their lives. When they can mark their own progress, they also find a sense of determination and perseverance.

Chapter 21
Study skills and homework

I had to train myself to focus my attention. I
became very visual and learned how to
create mental images in order to
comprehend what I read.

Tom Cruise, actor[98]

At school or university, studying and revising are important skills we need to acquire to test our ability and knowledge in certain topics or subjects regularly. No two people study the same way, but the aim is to ensure automatic recall of information. Study skills include researching information, taking notes, writing essays, revision and effective examination techniques. I believe study skills should be taught in primary school as soon as children are expected to sit tests and exams.

Most of us hate revising for tests and exams. Remember, many dyslexic learners may or may not suffer from short-term memory problems – information overload, organisation, attention, processing speed or sequencing problems may be issues too. Dyslexic learners feel overwhelmed when they don't know how to attack a whole year's-worth of information for several subjects and commit it all to memory. This is when avoidance tactics kick in.

If your child knows how to revise (which needs to be taught and doesn't come naturally), then he should be more willing and able to do it. Even when children reach university, they are overwhelmed by not knowing how to revise larger volumes of information. Being able to commit a year's-worth of topics to memory is vital to your child's success in school too, so it warrants having several sessions of study skills and being shown how to organise the material, use index and flash cards and work out which information is relevant to learn.

Perhaps the most important way to help your child is by being available to help him get organised. Encouraging him to find the discipline to spend time doing homework every day will set future expectations.

Memory and study skills: setting the stage

For dyslexic learners, remembering is a learned skill and, for children with dyslexia in particular, it is a hard-earned skill.

Learning to move information from short-term to long-term memory effectively is an important skill for studying. The word 'studying' implies concentrating on moving information into long-term memory to demonstrate mastery of a subject. There are ways to master the skill of memorisation and, with practice, your child can learn how to remember more effectively.

This section focuses on physical and mental strategies for improving memorisation. They include strategies, such as eating well so that you are not distracted by hunger, and standing up and walking around to keep yourself alert, to intellectual strategies such as setting a timer to limit study periods, and reducing distractions so that you can focus. For more information on memory learning techniques, see the **Memory and Memory Strategies** chapter.

Get in the zone

To set the stage for effective memorisation, we need to clear our minds, free ourselves of distraction and bring our concentration into focus. A good way to move information from your short-term to your long-term memory is by using your own powers of concentration. For some of us, this comes naturally. Others have to work harder at it. The techniques I suggest below are handy but, before you can employ them, you need to concentrate. Our powers of concentration are best when we are well rested, interested, 'tuned in' to what we are learning, and understand its purpose.

When great tennis players are focused on a game, you see them employ a number of tricks. From a distance, this looks like a series of nervous habits. They tug on their clothing or their hair, move the racquet from one hand to another and so on. If you watch the same player repeatedly, you will notice that this series of 'nervous habits' is the same every time. The player is getting in the zone. By performing the same series of moves every time, they are tuning in their brains and focusing. You can teach your child to do the same thing.

A simple habit, or sequence of rituals, performed in the same way every time you sit down to study will help you to tune in. Your brain quickly learns that, when this series of moves takes place, important learning is about to happen. Every child can create his own series of moves to get in the zone. It might be turning on the computer, sharpening a pencil and arranging his desk. Whatever it is, doing it the same way every day will make it an effective habit.

Take a break

A good way to prepare for effective memorisation is to set a timer or stopwatch. For reading passages, timing yourself works well. For memorising lists of numbers, dates, chemicals and so on, divide the work into logical sections and focus on one section at a time. Take a short mental break, then move on to the next section. After the second section, see what you recall from the first section. This will reinforce the learning. It helps to set aside a specific amount of time, say half an hour, on each activity. After that, do something different. If you have not memorised enough material in the allocated time, come back to it another day or later the same day. Always go over what you have already learned before moving on to the next part, to reinforce the learning.

Learning happens best in small quantities over short periods with frequent rests. Some of us have difficulty with the concept of taking breaks. It can feel like wasting precious time, time that should be better spent learning. Breaks can be short – five minutes every twenty to thirty minutes should do the trick – but the mental refreshment from the break is truly valuable and the bigger waste of time is sitting still poring over a book when the words have long since started to dance before our eyes and the text has lost all meaning.

Several short sessions of intense concentration with rests in between are more productive than one long session where you try to cram multiple facts into your head at once to get it over with.

It takes time for our brains to process new information, especially very unfamiliar information, such as a new way to solve a mathematical formula or a new period of history. Even if we are learning in an area that is familiar, it takes time for new information to sink in. Read something over and then take a break. Let your mind process something overnight, and come back to it the next day. After frequent repetition, unfamiliar information begins to sound familiar and new concepts are easier to understand through familiarity.

Get physical – get ready for learning

Sitting still and learning things can be hard work, especially for dyslexic learners, who tend to be creative and kinaesthetic, hands-on learners. It helps to take breaks and do some physical stretching or moving around, but why not combine learning with physical activity? Use your hands, stomp your feet, walk around the room or roll about on an exercise ball while you learn. It makes the activity more fun, alleviates the stress of sitting still, and makes remembering easier.

Educational kinesiology and Brain Gym

Educational kinesiology means learning through movement. All learning begins with movement of some kind. Reading uses eye movement, for example. Writing requires hand-to-eye coordination and fine motor skills. Brain Gym[99] is a form of kinesiology that consists of a set of movements that help right-brain thinkers use brain exercises to connect the left and right sides of their brain, helping them become more whole-brain thinkers. The Brain Gym® programme, developed by Dr Paul Dennison, an American Educational kinesiologist, has become popular throughout the world and is now used in over 80 countries, including the UK, North America and Australia. It is based on the theory that combining learning with the right set of movements will help to construct new pathways in the brain, leading to improved learning ability. It is often used to help people with dyslexia or learning difficulties improve their learning and coordination skills.

Brain Gym® uses 26 basic movements to assist learning and integrate mental learning with physical movement, thereby integrating mind and body. The movements are based on those we perform as babies and toddlers when we first learn motor skills and integrate the movements of our hands, ears, eyes and so on. The exercises are said to improve memory, concentration, physical coordination, organisational skills, and also reading, writing and maths skills.

Even though it is not clear why these movements work so well, teachers often report that they bring about improvements in areas such as concentration, focus, memory, coordination and learning skills. The movements help children relax, they find it fun and it prepares them for learning. Children generally have a big smile on their face when doing these fun exercises, especially when I drop the ball or mix up my left hand to right knee exercises!

The Primary Movement Programme[100]

The Primary Movement® programme (PMG) involves the daily repetition (10–15 minutes daily) of a short sequence of movements that mimic the early movements of a newborn child, the asymmetrical tonic neck reflex (ATNR) or 'fencing reflex'. The programme is presented in a child-friendly way in schools, with singing, actions, rhythms and exercises designed to stimulate the maturation of the central nervous system.

A study[101] conducted on 683 children found ATNR persistence and reported significant improvement in reading and Maths. The programme not only benefits children with reading, spelling and maths problems, but also those with coordination and handwriting problems, and is generally constructive fun for the whole school. Perhaps you could get your school involved in such a programme?

Exercise helps supply oxygen to the brain

We do know that any exercise increases oxygen to the brain, which is good for learning. Regardless of whether we are advocates of Brain Gym or the Primary Movement Programme, we know that exercise is critically important to brain function and memory. Researchers have found that exercise keeps the heart strong, the blood vessels open, and boosts blood supply, which in turn ensures that brain cells receive the nutrients they need for peak performance. Exercise helps supply oxygen to the brain, which makes the brain function better.

Any form of physical activity increases the flow of oxygen to the brain. Even walking 15 minutes a day to school will help your child focus better.

It's all in the timing

Many of us function better at certain times of day. The best time can be different for each of us. Some are night owls and some are early risers. People with dyslexia are especially prone to favour certain times of day when they feel at their peak. If possible, encourage your child to develop a habit of studying when he is at his peak. In my experience, children are fresher and more alert in the morning. By the time they come home from school, they are exhausted from having to concentrate twice as hard to remember information as a child who does not have learning difficulties.

Successful study environment

For dyslexic learners, studying, especially academic studying, is hard work. Many will naturally fight against it and be unwilling to embrace it. Setting up a comfortable home environment is vital to success. There are three essential ingredients to a successful study environment. It doesn't have to be fancy, but look around your home or your child's bedroom and see if you can find a corner that satisfies these three points:

1. Comfortable

2. Organised

3. Free from distraction

Successful Study Environment

Comfortable. Lighting needs to be good, seating should be comfortable and a flat surface for writing on and spreading out study aids. This could be a desk with a lamp, a low level table and a cushion on the floor, or whatever makes your child comfortable. It need not be traditional and it's okay if your child wants to listen to gentle background music while he works. One good idea is to keep a couple of favourite things around (a cherished photo, favourite instrument or special souvenir).

Organised. You may need to help your child create and maintain an organised space. Some people with dyslexia are not good at organising. If your child fits this category, it's okay to help him organise his materials and tidy them up periodically so that they are easy to find. The trick is to minimise distractions and keep him focused on the homework task at hand.

Before beginning a learning session, make sure your child has all his things around him: books, pencils, paper, index cards, high lighters, scissors, glue or whatever he needs to accomplish his learning effectively. It is one thing taking a break, but quite another being continuously distracted or unable to concentrate because he is bobbing up and down looking for the supplies he needs.

Free from distraction. People with dyslexia need peace and quiet to focus. While it might be okay to listen to some light music in the background, it is not okay if the space is constantly interrupted by other family members or unwanted distractions such as the TV blaring in the background - keep TV for the reward after homework is done. Likewise, if something more exciting is going on in another part of the house, it will be hard for your child to focus. Try to create a consistent time each day when the whole household has settled down into quiet activities and stillness has descended on the home.

Our homework place was in the kitchen. My children generally started their homework while I was preparing supper, and were able to spread out their work on the table while I was cooking. I was close at hand and available for questions, but I didn't sit watching over them unless they needed help with something specific. That was how we both maximised our time, and I didn't feel I was just sitting there with nothing to do when they didn't need me.

Another natural place for doing homework might be around the computer. If so, make the computer area cosy. Don't banish the computer to a remote nook in the attic or a cold corner of the basement. Most children prefer to feel part of the family area when they are doing their homework. It's almost that feeling of not wanting to miss out on what is going on, plus feeling supported.

Establish a routine

I can't emphasise enough how important it is to establish a routine. Remember that keyword 'automaticity'. When you do something often and regularly, it becomes ingrained in your brain and you feel lost without it. Workaholics, when robbed of the opportunity to do overtime, often feel unanchored and don't know how to spend their free time. That's because their minds are locked in to working all day and they have developed a strong habit of doing so. I am not suggesting that you turn your child into a homework-aholic, but consistent routine that occurs at a set time each day will help lock in his brain, so that he is ready to work at that time. He will come to the table more prepared and willing, subconsciously as well as consciously, to take on his homework. Little and often is preferable to our memory than cramming in one session.

I do not believe, however, in cracking the whip. I would get better results from my children if I encouraged strongly rather than forcing or insisting. The more fun you can make it, the more willingly your child will approach the task. It is hard to be creative and patient all the time, and it is hard to give of your time to help your child on a consistent basis. Starting to see the rewards of your work will encourage you to keep it up.

Don't forget to allow time for breaks, and schedule the homework time to allow for any extra-curricular activities your child enjoys. There are times when they won't seem to have much homework and others when the going seems brutal.

I use a selection of motivational and getting-organised charts to encourage my children and help them manage their own learning. There are some examples in the Appendix.

Developing concentration

Maintaining concentration is often a problem when you have to do something you find difficult or hate. For dyslexic learners, it can be hard to concentrate on both reading and writing. It is more difficult to tune out distractions when they are not enjoying what they are doing. Try and look for ways to make the task more enjoyable. Earlier I talked about the importance of setting up a comfortable workspace, free from distractions. Encourage them to study in short bursts, taking time in between to freshen up.

Concentration is also easier if your physiological needs have been met: quality sleep, good food and physical exercise. Then, it will be easier for him to focus when he needs to sit still and apply himself.

When your child sits down to study, encourage him to set a goal for that study session, and stop when he meets it. If his mind starts to wander, encourage him to bring it back to the goal. If he meets the goal ahead of schedule, congratulate him and suggest that he enjoy the extra time. That makes it easier to sit down next time.

When you get stuck

Sometimes, no matter how hard we study, we just get stuck. This becomes a major distraction and demotivator. When your child gets stuck, encourage him to spend a few minutes reviewing the problem. Can someone help him read over his notes? Is the answer in his textbook and he just cannot find it? Can someone help him find where to look in his textbook? After a few minutes, if he still cannot find the answer, suggest that he stop working on that problem and turn to something else. Sometimes, our brains need time away from a problem.

Often, as we let something sit in the back of our mind, the answer becomes apparent, but sometimes we need to work through a problem in detail, step by step, to analyse it or discover the solution. Maths problems fall into this category. They can't be solved by reading the maths book. Your child needs to study with a pencil and paper, and work through the examples systematically until he understands them. After several attempts, he could make a note to ask his teacher the next day and then move on.

Managing homework

Homework and revising are frustrating chores for most children. For children with dyslexia, homework time can be an upsetting period for the whole family. It can tug at your heart strings to watch your child wrestle with a frustrating homework task. At the same time, it will gnaw at your patience when it takes countless attempts to remember a simple fact that is forgotten the next day.

Remember that a homework assignment is to practise and reinforce something your child has just learned in school.

Children may need help with reading and understanding the assignment itself. You may need to help him read and interpret the task and then go over it several times until he grasps it. Help your child break the task into small chunks to get started and encourage him to do quality work on one assignment at a time rather than rush through the tasks to get them over with. You can draw pictures or Mind Maps® as you go to make it easier for him to visualise the assignment as well as hear or read it. For a complex task such as writing an essay, you may need to help him develop an overall plan for it.

One problem you will probably run into repeatedly is the forgotten homework syndrome. Your child will frustrate you by forever forgetting the required textbook, homework assignment sheet or even leaving his entire book bag at school. Encourage him to keep a homework diary or calendar book and write down everything – ask the teacher to check it before he leaves school. If writing down the assignment is frustrating, encourage him to make an oral note, perhaps by investing in an inexpensive recording device (some are small enough to fit on a key ring). A teacher may be able to leave a voice note so you can hear the teacher's instructions for yourself.

When your child has finished a homework task, check that he has fulfilled the instructions. Is the essay within the required word count? Has he completed all the assigned maths problems? Does the history timeline cover the required dates and capture the essential historical milestones? Perform a check on spelling and look over the work to ensure that it is legible. This is very important with maths assignments. Teachers can't give a mark to illegible answers.

Some schools now post online information such as homework assignments, project timescales, due-in dates and revision materials. If your school runs a website, try and become familiar with it and look at it regularly with your child to make sure you are up to date with assignments. Make a note of the teachers who don't post notes regularly and stay in touch with them a different way.

Planning writing assignments for older children

A way to break a blank piece of paper is simply to start writing whatever comes into your head. But don't let your child do this! It is important to plan the work before starting to write. Planning will save your child time and energy.

Encourage your child to take five minutes to plan each essay or story, even if he is in a hurry. Planning pays huge dividends. It forces him to think the process through logically (beginning, middle and end) and makes him consider his end result or conclusion. Once he has jotted a few ideas on paper (either list or Mind Map®), it becomes easier to see what to write about. Sometimes it helps to start thinking about the conclusion first and work backwards. Using a computer makes it much easier to edit.

The Planning Writing Assignments table will help your child understand the order of planning an assignment.

Planning Writing Assignments

Organisation: Make a plan. For example, plan how much time you need to do background research on the topic, then make time to assemble the research and develop an essay plan. Finally, plan how long you need to write. Don't forget you need time to proof read.

Time Management: Set yourself a schedule and try to stick to it. After you have pored over a single paragraph for ten minutes, leave it and come back to it later rather than stare at it or reword it over and over.

Plan your Essay: Take five minutes to Mind Map® or list the points you want to make and then make sure you make them.

References: Always remember to acknowledge your sources when your ideas or quotes come from other works. There is nothing wrong with expressing someone else's idea as long as you give them credit.

Plagiarism: Plagiarism is checked for in most schools using online computer programmes that scan your essay and look for matches in other online articles. Make sure you rewrite everything in your own words and give due credit to other authors when you use their ideas.

Proofread: Leave at least five minutes at the end of your work or exam to proofread your work. You may gain as much as 10% in marks by checking your working through.

Spelling and Grammar: If you are using a computer programme enlarge the view to 100% or more. Usual spellcheckers do not help people with dyslexia, **Ginger** software spelling and grammar check is very helpful for individuals with dyslexia. Check for sentences that are too long (hint: too many commas in a single sentence is a sign that you need to break it into two shorter ones or sentences that are more than a few lines long). Get someone to proof read it with you.

Punctuation: Check that you have used capital letters after full stops, commas, speech marks, brackets, exclamation and question marks. Check you have used paragraphs.

Sense: Does your work make sense? Most computer programmes don't check for this, although Ginger software is pretty good at finding grammatical and syntax errors. If possible, get someone to read it through for you.

Reading for information

If your child wants to study effectively, it helps to keep in the forefront of his mind exactly what he is trying to accomplish.

Good questions to ask before starting to read a text are: 'Why am I reading this? What is it I need to find out?' His approach to the reading should be different depending on his objective. Is he revising for an exam? Learning about a new subject? Comparing the author's viewpoint to that of another author? If he is writing an essay, he needs first to make an essay plan, and then plan the main points. The introduction should introduce the argument he wishes to make in the essay and the conclusion sums up his main points. The paragraphs in between need to discuss his ideas about the subject, build the argument that supports his final conclusion, and support his argument with references or examples.

There is not just one speed for reading. If your child is learning something new, for example, he might prefer to read slowly and even read out loud to give himself time to absorb the new information. Or he might need to scan the material to highlight keywords and read more in depth when he finds a keyword he is looking for. If the material is new and it is important he learns it, he should take notes as he reads to refer back to later as a concise summary of what he needs to learn. If reading for him is difficult, he can use text to speech software or a reading pen.

I always ask children to read any comprehension questions first, then highlight the key phrases or words they feel are important in answering the questions. In this way, the child gets a good feel for the information he is about to read, and the brain will notice the key phrases when he reads the text.

There are various techniques for reading and all serve different purposes. Share these with your child:

Reading for Information

Active reading: Make notes while reading, read out loud, or record yourself reading and play it back to yourself later to reinforce what you learned.

Rapid reading: Read quickly through something to recall key points and ideas, or locate important information that you want to read in more detail.

Scanning: Skim your eyes over the written page to isolate keywords or key phrases, dates and so on. This helps you zoom in quickly on specific information you are looking for when you don't want to read the whole article or text.

Reading instructions: This is particularly important if you are taking an exam or preparing for an essay. Read through the instructions slowly and carefully and repeat back to yourself (in your mind) what you have just read. Make sure you have understood the instructions exactly. If you are not sure, take a deep breath in and out, then read it again. Highlight key words and write any word numbers as numerals alongside, e.g. 'Answer three (3) questions in full'. The eye will 'see' the number 3 better and you won't be tempted to misread and write two or four answers.

SQ3R[102] is a reading technique for understanding and remembering material you read. It consists of five steps:

Survey – (1 minute) Quickly scan headings and sub-headings.

Question – (30 seconds) Ask yourself, 'What is this chapter about?'

Read – (might be slow for dyslexic learners – this is active reading). Read one section at a time.

Recite/write – (1 minute) Say aloud to reinforce and make notes of key phrases.

Review – (10 minutes) After reading each chapter, your child will have a list of key phrases from steps 2–4 that provide an outline/summary for each chapter. He can test himself by covering the key phrases and trying to recall them (you

> might help). It is best to try to reproduce any diagrams or tables that are relevant examples. If he cannot remember one of his major points, he needs to reread that section

When the reading material is particularly difficult, or your child is finding it difficult to remember what he is reading, he could try skimming it first a couple of times to pick out some salient points, and highlight key phrases or draw a picture in the margin to 'visualise' what he has read. Then he can go back and begin reading again, this time more slowly, and try to connect the dots in his mind from one salient point to the next.

If there is a passage he just does not understand, try and read it out loud. If he still does not get it, he could try skipping over it to see if he can pick up what he needs to learn from the next few paragraphs. Tell him not to be discouraged if he cannot pick up the thread throughout every paragraph for an entire chapter. He will probably assimilate enough information from the paragraphs he can understand to compensate for the part he missed.

Taking notes in class

Taking effective notes is an important skill, especially in classes where the teacher stands at the front and lectures. Good note-taking is important for when children have to do homework assignments – children need to be able to read and understand what they have written.

Note-taking can be troublesome for dyslexic learners who cannot write as fast as the teacher is talking or read back what they have written. A good tip is to divide every page with a vertical straight line one third of the way down the page. On the left-hand side, your child can write down the main ideas, and on the right-hand side as many details as possible, using abbreviations and short sentences. It isn't necessary to write down everything the teacher is saying, but just enough to jog the memory when going over the notes later. Then, the visual separation between the main ideas and the details will help him construct an essay plan or find the part of the lesson he wishes to review.

If your child struggles with taking notes in class, I suggest asking his teacher to record the session if possible, and to ask for hand outs of class or lecture notes. Sometimes, it is difficult to take in what is being said while writing speed notes at the same time, especially for someone who isn't an auditory learner.

Giving presentations in front of the class

Talking in front of the class can be nerve wracking for anyone. The key to overcoming nerves is to be organised and plan the presentation really well. Index cards are a good way to organise thoughts. They don't have to have words on them; symbols or images can be used as memory joggers.

When watching other people presenting, it will become clear that a good presentation depends just as much on the personality of the presenter as it does on the information being presented. Your child may not read as quickly as some of his peers, but children with dyslexia can be personable and charming, with much personality. If he infuses his presentation with humour and looks the audience in the eye, he will engage his audience.

Before giving the presentation, your child needs to rehearse how to stand and where to put his hands. It is okay to hold his hands gently folded in front of him or to make gestures, or to keep one hand neatly tucked in a pocket – but he needs to be careful not to jingle change or keys, as that is a sign of nerves. Some people like to hold something (a pen or a pointer, index cards), but the distracting sound of clicking a ballpoint pen on and off is not a good idea! The trick is to look relaxed, even though he may not feel it.

Two more common mistakes people make are (1) talking so fast that people cannot absorb what is being said and (2) forgetting to explain topics adequately so that people are able follow. So he needs to remember to slow down, take time to explain concepts that might be new to others, and ask if anyone has any questions at the end.

By the way, if someone asks a question to which he does not know the answer, he can thank them for asking a great question, then ask the audience if anyone would like to answer that one – someone might and then he is off the hook, gracefully! If no one knows, he can answer with good humour that he is now curious and will look the answer up later.

Revision strategies

Studying, learning and memorising are all essentially tied together to form the act of acquiring new information in a permanent area of the brain so that it can be recalled at will and used when needed. I have talked at length throughout this book about memorisation and the three magic words:

Repetition, repetition, repetition

Repetition and practice are key revision strategies. Having easy access to revision notes and well laid-out and organised notes is essential if your child is going to review information regularly. I recommend having a separate revision exercise book, so that individual pieces of paper are not lost or screwed up. Your child may need to memorise the same or similar information over a couple of years or more, and will be able to pick up his condensed revision notes already prepared and keep adding new material when it needs to be revised, which will save much time and effort. Share the summary table of revision strategies with your child.

Revision Strategies
Know Your VAK Learning Style and Multiple Intelligences: Knowing how your brain learns best is an essential foundation for revising.
Get Enough Sleep: A tired brain cannot learn effectively. If you are tired, get some sleep and return to studying when you are rested. This is also true if you are angry, sad or preoccupied emotionally. Go for a walk or a quick jog, take some deep breaths in the fresh air or meditate, and then come back to your studies in a calmer state.
Revision Timetable: Make a weekly revision chart with the subjects you will study each day and tick them off so you can see your progress.

Be Realistic: Know how much you can accomplish in one day and be realistic about it. If you have multiple subjects for exam week, start revising early – do not leave it to the week before. Manage your time!

Make it a Habit: Study every day at the same time, and develop a ritual for getting started. This makes it easier to sit down and study every day. Mornings are the best.

Short Sessions: Learning happens best in short spurts. Experts suggest having a break every 20-30 minutes – get up, walk around, have a glass of water to re-energise, and then recap what you have just learned before you start the next topic.

Revise Often: When learning very complex material, don't just learn it once. Studies show that you are much more likely to retain information if you reinforce what you have learned and review it several times over several days than if you cram for one day and never return to it.

Drink Water: Your brain needs water and oxygen to optimise its performance.

Do Something Fun: In your revision timetable, include doing something fun every day!

Don't Give Up! You can do this. Keep your motivation high. Read inspirational stories of people doing what you would like to do in life and be encouraged. All things worth having require strength and perseverance.

Strategies for exam taking

You may think that exams are about the worst thing that can happen to your child, but don't despair. Before getting into exam-taking tips, let me just say that, whenever possible, look for courses that put emphasis on grading work throughout the course, rather than being weighted towards the final exams. This is not always possible at the secondary- or high-school level, but is definitely an option at college or university.

Talk over the following table of Exam Tips with your child.

Exam Tips

Don't skip classes. Attend all available classes, including the last one or two prior to the exam so you can glean every last point and exam tips.

Make sure you understand the format of the exam before you take it and whether it will be multiple choice, written answers, etc. Teachers will have gone through old exam papers, ask for more past papers and review them at home. Identify how much time you will need for each section and try to absorb the general instructions for the exam before you go into the exam room.

Prepare mentally. Revise well in advance, not the night before an exam. Review key notes again the day before.

Get a study buddy. Go over the material out loud with a friend and bounce ideas off each other about what the test will be like.

Make a written list of equipment you are allowed to bring into the exam (pencils, calculator, etc.) and check them off the list before you leave home. Place the list somewhere you will see it, such as on the front door or on the breakfast table.

Go to bed early the night before the exam and arrive early to give you time to get in the zone.

When you take the exam, look over the whole exam paper and verify whether it is what you were expecting. Identify any hard spots and leave them until last.

Watch the clock and manage your time well. If you have extra time, decide how you are going to best use it. Try to stay within the time constraints for each section so that you are able to complete the exam. Write down how many minutes you are going to spend on each question, taking into consideration the marks per question. Highlight the questions you need to answer, so that you don't miss them out.

Focus first on the areas that are easiest for you and the areas worth the most points. Return to the harder parts at the end, as time allows.

For essay questions take 5 minutes to make a brief essay plan, then follow it. This helps you to focus and not lose your train of thought. Sometimes exam papers ask you to do this on the answer paper. Write your brief plan at the beginning of your essay, listing the main points in a few bullets. This tells the examiner what you planned to say even if you accidentally miss out the points or run out of time.

Do not leave multiple choice questions unanswered. There is generally no penalty for a wrong answer. Use guesswork to answer any questions to which you don't know the answer. Statistics for multiple-choice test-taking show that the odds are in a student's favour for guessing answers even if penalties for wrong answers are applied.

Try to write clearly so that your answers are legible even though you are nervous and trying to concentrate on the material.

Leave five minutes in reserve to review and proofread your writing for spelling, grammar, punctuation and that it makes sense. It can mean the difference between a marginal pass or fail, or going up a grade.

Remember the admin basics. Make sure you have put your name or any identifying information (such as a student ID number) on your paper.

Stay positive

Your attitude will greatly influence your child's attitude. Children are very intuitive. It is vital that you maintain a belief in the fact that your son or daughter can succeed in life despite their dyslexia. Praise every triumph, sympathise with every disaster, but don't let them give up or give up on them.

Remind them that persistence and dedication are valuable assets. Make sure they don't leave homework and revising to the last minute. By being methodical and organised in their approach, they should have every expectation of attaining the educational level they want to achieve.

— ✧ —

PART SIX
Your Young Adult

Chapter 22
Learning how to drive

I don't like driving very much. That makes me
very unhappy, because I scream a lot in the
car, but other than that, life is actually pretty
good.

Whoopi Goldberg, actress[103]

We all want to pass our driving test first time round. There is
kudos attached to doing that. Many teenagers who do
not have dyslexia don't pass first time, but if your child has
dyslexia or a learning difficulty, he may have a harder time
learning how to drive and passing the test, depending on his
areas of strength and weakness.

Both my children took a while to learn how to drive. My
daughter found the multitasking aspect of driving quite
daunting. She also said that trying to remember all the theory
test signs was difficult: 'It's tricky for a dyslexic person to
remember what the no stopping sign means!' My son found the
mechanics of driving and parking straightforward, but said that
his visual perception (his own words!) and gauging distances
were tricky for him.

Both youngsters felt pressure because their friends had
passed quickly, but they took much longer. I suggested having
as many driving lessons as possible, and to sit or retake the test
only when *they* were ready, and not to compare themselves to
their friends. They were frustrated at having to depend on other
people to get them around and disappointed that they found
driving difficult.

If your teenager has been formally diagnosed with a
specific learning difficulty, you will know from his educational

assessment report what his challenges are. Problems in the following areas may make learning to drive more challenging:

- visual perceptual
- sequencing instructions
- remembering left from right
- reading maps and signs
- instruction overload
- hand-to-eye coordination skills
- background noises
- reaction time
- remembering lots of theory data
- attention.

Some people with dyslexia have perceptual problems. However, many others have strengths in the areas of spatial awareness, spatial relationships or hand-to-eye coordination. So don't assume that your child will have problems. If you already know your child has perceptual problems, he may receive information inaccurately through his senses and have trouble processing it, because the information becomes confused as it travels from his eyes or ears to the brain.

It may take some dyslexic learners longer than the average time to develop automatic skills in driving. They may have to concentrate harder. For example, they may not be able to talk to a passenger at the same time as driving. If your child is still having problems remembering left and right, he will find following or receiving left/right instructions difficult, but there are ways around this problem. When practising, he can have a picture showing left and right and the words on the dashboard. He may also find looking in the mirror and seeing behind him confusing and disorientating.

In the UK, the theory test takes 40 minutes, but a person with dyslexia can have double that time – up to 80 minutes. When applying to take the test, he needs to ask for extra time and present a report or letter from a psychologist or specialist teacher. The theory test also has the option for dyslexic candidates to listen to the test being read in English or in 20 other languages.

As with any other topic, driving theory should be presented in small, manageable chunks. In order to remember all the information, it can be presented using VAK methods such as visual or audio CDs and, of course, plenty of practical driving experience. Your child can use revision strategies and memorisation techniques, just as for memorising any type of information.

Find an instructor who is an expert at teaching dyslexic learners and ask for extra time in the theory test. A step-by-step, slow approach is the best one.

Chapter 23
Further education and careers advice: late teens and young adults

> School gave me a fundamental
> understanding of what I was not good at. It
> gave me an acute desire to find something,
> a life preserver, and I found swimming.
>
> *Duncan Goodhew, Olympic swimmer*[104]

If your child was not diagnosed as having dyslexia until his teen years, or he has already left school, you may well feel that the system has failed him, and you would be right. If your child has slipped through the net or has not been given the care he should have received, he may have left school with few or no qualifications. Please do not despair. You may both have gone through hell if this is the case; but there is hope and there are still opportunities open to him.

At the end of this chapter, I provide an overview of opportunities that exist for older children and young adults with dyslexia in different English-speaking countries. My goal is to make you aware there are plenty of options, and to provide you with some resources to spur your own search for opportunities in your local area. It is never too late to be tested, diagnosed or to find help. If you even suspect dyslexia in your older child at this point, press on and arrange for a proper evaluation or free careers assessment. You will be glad you did.

My daughter really wanted to go to university and be treated the same as the rest of her friends. She entered university through what would once have been considered an atypical route. After leaving school at 16, she knew she didn't want to continue studying academic subjects in depth, so I encouraged her to pursue topics she loved: acting, singing or using her incredible people skills. The reason she left her school was because the choices were very narrow and mostly academic (and boring, to my mind). Had I insisted on her studying academic subjects that were on offer, or even business studies, she would have been miserable. So she went to college and first began a two-year course in photography, theatre studies and media studies.

Unfortunately, there was still a fair amount of theory attached to these subjects, which she found a challenge but, with help, she passed the first-year exams. Thereafter, she realised that acting wasn't her thing and changed to a music and singing course that was half practical based, and half exam based. The hands-on style of learning suited her, but she still found the written exams tricky.

She passed her music course but felt the competition was too great to become a 'star', and that she wanted to concentrate on her other strengths – her people skills. So she applied to several universities for Events Management, with her accumulated 'exam points'. She was offered an unconditional place by one university and two other conditional places, and she went off to university. Finally, she felt the same as the rest of her friends. Leaving home, off to university to experience what many teenagers are dying to do.

Another assessment had to be done for university so that she could continue to be allowed extra time in exams and dyslexia support, and be entitled to the DSA (Disabled Students' Allowance) that universities offer to those with learning difficulties.

Even though the course was mostly project-based, which was better for her than the stress of exams, many of the assignments required linking events and marketing theory to real-life tasks. So, my daughter asked me for guidance with some of her assignments that involved extensive reading and having to quote and reference theory.

The second year was an internship in an events organisation. She found a job in the sailing events world and, finally, had found her passion. They loved her at work, and she was brilliant at managing big events and people, networking, selling and building up business contacts.

Towards the end of her internship, she said she needed to talk to me... I had already expected that she would not want to go back to university to complete her degree. She wanted confirmation and acceptance from me and her dad that we supported her decision to stay in the working world. And we did.

The message here is: allow your children to follow their heart and their dreams. Sometimes these dreams don't work out, but they need to find this out for themselves. If they are making very unwise decisions due to lack of experience, we can show them all the options and review the pros and cons with them, but making children do something they don't feel good at, or don't have a strength in, may hold them back from discovering their true vocation.

Today's world offers a wide range of higher education opportunities, without necessarily having to go to university.

There are dedicated technical schools that train students for specific jobs such as dental hygienist, car mechanic, aviation technician, veterinarian assistant, legal secretary, hairdressing and many other excellent vocations. There is also a multitude of online classes offered by both obscure and highly recognised universities. Trade and vocational schools and colleges (also called Career Colleges in Canada) and online classes and e-learning are available to everybody, but may be particularly helpful to dyslexic students.

Vocation/trade schools often use hands-on training methods and focus less on written academic work. Online classes allow students to go at their own pace, so they are not measuring themselves against others in the class, and have time to stop and think, plan their writing assignments and so on.

Careers advice

Before teenagers can decide which course is right for their career path, they need to identify which career direction is right for them. Some young people may feel that they have plenty of time ahead of them but, if your child is over 15, I suggest having careers advice as soon as possible. It will guide him to make the right subject choices at secondary level as well as for further education.

The UK government offers free careers advice at **nationalcareersservice.direct.gov.uk** with coaching professionals who can offer advice on choosing the right course, identifying strengths and abilities, creating a CV, and interview skills.

Morrisby is a private organisation that undertakes paid assessments to establish career options **www.morrisby.com**. It is a comprehensive analysis of an individual's abilities, interests, learning styles and personality. The purpose is to match career choices to courses and to present suggestions. The report also gives advice on work experience, gap years and personal development plans.

A career assessment will give your older child a better understanding of himself. It often makes people think about issues they had not previously considered. For example, when considering a career or job, it is not only the nature of the work that is important, but also the working environment. It is often the first time that teenagers have thought about themselves in this way, and this self-knowledge is crucial in helping them make informed decisions about their future. Do they like working under pressure, lots of admin and report writing, or can they handle strict deadlines? These elements may have a bearing on whether a job might be more or less suitable. It makes them think whether they have the right personality for a particular type of work.

A career assessment may identify significant abilities and talents teenagers didn't realise they had

The preferred learning styles analysis is particularly useful when discussing where students want to go and what they want to study. This is particularly helpful as methods of assessment can vary depending on whether your child follows the traditional university degree route or a more vocational route. If he finds it hard to learn facts, or goes to pieces during exams, he certainly does not want to take a course where the outcome depends entirely on exams! For children with learning difficulties who have struggled in the school system or who were never identified as having dyslexia or special needs, the assessment may identify significant abilities and talents they didn't realise they had.

**A career assessment may identify dyslexia
or special needs not picked up at school**

Online versus onsite education

Today's world makes it possible for us to experience education online so that we can fit it into our busy lives. But there is so much extra that you learn when you attend in person and interact with different instructors with different methods of instruction, witness their perspectives, get their personal vibes and hear their stories. You also have the opportunity to interact with other learners.

In many cases, over half the learning experience takes place when you hear the stories and experiences of other students who are there to learn, but have much to teach, especially at the level of adult education. They will have trodden different paths from yourself, so can help to broaden your horizons and give you a range of insights at different levels across your subject area that a single instructor cannot give. Going to school or college as a young or older adult is a very different experience from what you go through as a child.

Online learning offers the possibility of education to those who otherwise would not be able to take classes, but, if you have the opportunity, I recommend attending in person for at least part of the time.

Finding out at university/college that your young adult has dyslexia

You would think that by the time your child had made it to university, you would know whether he had a learning difficulty or not. Unfortunately, this is not always the case.

Every day, teenagers and young adults find out that they have dyslexia or a specific learning difficulty and are not coping well at college or university. If their learning difficulty is not picked up, some drop out because they cannot cope. They would be able to manage had they been previously identified with a learning difficulty and received the right level of support in their first year.

Discovering relatively late that you have dyslexia can be a shattering experience or a great relief. Many young adults go through a rollercoaster of emotions, from relief to anger and back again, which can last for some time. Your child's response depends on his ability and level of maturity to be able to manage this unfamiliar situation.

Take time out to discuss what exactly your child is finding tough

Even when our children become young adults, they may still turn to us for help (we hope). If your teenager or young adult is struggling at university in spite of achieving good or high grades to get in, then assuming he is not burning the midnight oil and partying every night, it is worth taking time out to discuss what exactly he is finding so tough. It is very important for your child to have access to sympathetic and practical support both at home and at university.

Get your teenager or young adult to ask if there is a mentoring scheme at university with second- or third-year students on the same course who have been in the same situation and can offer practical advice. That way he could have more contact with other dyslexic students. Or ask if there is a Q&A session where he can ask questions from second-year students in the year above – students relate better to other students and are more likely to accept advice from a peer than an adult. If a support structure doesn't exist – create it! Be the one who changes the system.

More often than not, teenagers do not want to lose face at university nor want their parents to worry, and generally they may not share their problem of not coping until it is too late. The worst situation is for those teenagers or young adults who do not have support from their families or have left home in a storm and no longer have contact with their family. These young adults have few people they feel able to turn to.

There is no question that university is a massive step up from secondary school. You are on your own in terms of independent learning. You are not spoon-fed, as you might be in a cosy classroom; you are left to research on your own and to read vast quantities of information, books and journals you have never encountered before. Then, you have to prioritise and interpret huge amounts of information and write coherent reports based on theory. Not easy!

Lectures are a difficult medium for learning for dyslexic students. Traditionally, lectures are auditory affairs to a large audience, with non-interactive visual slides that involve little audience participation, with the exception of group assignments. There is also a lot of note-taking. When students take notes, they cannot take in what is being said. If their note-taking ends up being illegible or they've omitted chunks of information, it is unlikely to make sense to them afterwards. Also, lectures are generally one-off topics that aren't repeated and reinforced as in school.

Students also face the problem of not being explicitly taught how to research. This is an art that takes time and experience to learn, and students generally aren't taught how to do this high level of research in secondary school, as most of the information they need to memorise is given in the curriculum. It seems that many are not explicitly shown how to do this in university either.

Teenagers are also not used to extended-essay writing and are not given templates to follow or examples of excellent pieces of work. At school, they have the opportunity to write, receive feedback and rewrite before they are graded. At university, they may have to submit work without prior feedback.

Another problem is the lack of close supervision teenagers benefited from in secondary school, and regular access to personal tutors. Many universities do assign tutors to students, but the tutor might be caring for many students and cannot give the same close supervision your teenager received at school.

Suddenly, the problems associated with dyslexia and learning difficulties, such as auditory learning, organisational skills, sequencing tasks and events, reading and remembering vast amounts of information, and a lack of kinaesthetic learning, rear their ugly heads. Repetition of key information is unlikely.

I believe there is a need for teaching at school of more independent learning and how to research and interpret information well. Being able to decipher what is relevant and irrelevant information is an art, and it takes a long time to acquire this skill. Dyslexic students don't always realise that they need not read every single word, which is an overwhelming task.

So what is the longer-term solution for universities helping non-diagnosed children who have dyslexia?

I suggest that it would make sense for the body that processes applications (UCAS in the UK) to ask students to complete the Lucid Adult Dyslexia Screening test (LADS), which takes only 20 minutes to administer, plus a simple learning styles questionnaire, or the Stamford Test or Centigrade Online as part of the application process (see more under the UCAS section, above), to establish if there are any learning challenges.

These courses of action will not only identify non-diagnosed dyslexia, they will also establish if teenagers are applying for the right course for them. Then, when they start university, they can receive from the outset the much-needed support on offer to diagnosed dyslexic students (see **Disabled Students' Allowance**). In the long run, it would reduce the dropout rate and save universities and governments huge amounts of money. Failing at university is a blow to young adults' self-esteem – a blow from which it takes a long time to recover.

Exciting work is not only possible – you should expect it!

Doing meaningful, rewarding work adds joy and purpose to our life. If you are not in the right career field, or stuck in a job where you are not fulfilling your potential, then the chances are you are finding life unrewarding, and often downright depressing. It is no way to live, and it is how people burn out.

When you find a job you love, which draws on your unique talents and strengths and makes you feel that you are contributing something useful in the world, everything looks brighter and feels better, and you are happy to get out of bed in the morning. We are all made to do something. Each of us brings something unique to this world. Do not focus on the talents you do not have. Focus instead on the talents you do have (hint: these are probably closely aligned with things you *like* doing).

If you want a degree, pursue one. There are many ways an adult or older child can find support for learning difficulties in higher education, and so many role models and examples of successful dyslexic students being teachers, lawyers, even writers. Options are everywhere. But you need to be motivated and determined to succeed.

On the other hand, not all of us are cut out for higher or further education, and would prefer to look for paid employment. Rather than get caught up in worrying about whether your child has the right number of school qualifications or a bachelor's degree, discuss with him what he really enjoys doing and wants to do (or not do) for the rest of his life. This should guide his education strategy rather than the need to tread the traditional path and do what everybody else did or does. There are many options; encourage him not to be disheartened and not to stop looking for rewarding work and a fulfilling career. Adults are less likely to burn out from doing a job they love.

United Kingdom further education options

If your older child is either thinking about going to university to do a degree or follow a vocational route, or has finished university and doesn't know what to do next it is a good idea to get careers advice.

Prospects[105] is an excellent organisation that provides careers advice, course information and job opportunities to students and postgraduates in the UK, plus information for students wanting to work abroad, with country-specific information about 80 countries for graduates searching for job opportunities after university.

Learn Direct[106] also provides excellent information about apprenticeships, courses and qualifications.

UCAS (Universities and Colleges Admission Service)

UCAS is the organisation responsible for managing applications to higher education courses in the UK **www.ucas.com**. If your child wants to go to university or college, he needs to know what qualifications and 'tariff points' are required to secure a place on an undergraduate course. Many different qualifications are covered by the UCAS tariff system; you can check the list on its website to see whether the course your teenager is considering is covered under the UCAS system.[107]

Your teenager also needs to know which topics interest him. There is helpful information on the UCAS website to help him identify his interests and abilities. There are a couple of questionnaires to help students match their interests and abilities to possible higher-education subjects.

The shorter questionnaire, the Stamford Test, is free, or there is a longer questionnaire, Centigrade Online **www.coa.co.uk**, that goes into greater detail, matching interests, study subjects and qualifications, and produces a unique report containing a selection of up to eight higher-education course areas based on your child's interests and abilities. Centigrade Online takes about half an hour to complete and is reasonably priced.

Many students find these online tests helpful even if they choose to go down a vocational route.

Disabled Students' Allowance (DSA)

Undergraduate, full-time, part-time and postgraduate students can apply for Disabled Students' Allowances[108], which are grants to help meet the extra course costs students can face as a direct result of a disability or specific learning difficulty such as dyslexia.

They are aimed at helping disabled people to study on an equal basis with other students. The amount paid doesn't depend on household income. DSAs are paid on top of the standard student finance package, and don't have to be paid back. The DSA can help pay for specialist equipment needed for studying, for example: computer software; a non-medical helper such as a note-taker or reader; extra travel costs necessary because of your disability; and other costs such as tapes, photocopying or Braille paper.

Bachelor's degree versus BTEC Higher Nationals (QCF)

A bachelor's degree is typically a three- or four-year university programme and much more academic in nature. Some degrees offer a sandwich year option too (a year out in industry).

BTEC Higher Nationals (HN)[109] are specialist vocational learning courses at Levels 4 or 5. There are around 40 industry sectors to choose from. There are full-time and part-time courses (meaning you can work as well). The BTEC Level 4 (Higher National Certificate) takes around two years part-time to complete; and the Level 5 (Higher National Diploma) is mainly a full-time course of study. They are an attractive option for students who may not be ready to do a degree. Once the HN is completed, it can lead to entry on the final year of a degree course.

NVQ and competence based qualifications (QCF)[110]

National Vocational Qualifications (NVQs) are delivered in the workplace or environments that replicate the workplace. Young adults are able to gain real hands-on experience at the same time as getting a qualification, and this may suit those who dislike examinations.

An NVQ demonstrates that an individual has both the knowledge and technical skills needed to do the job. There are over 90 different industry sectors to choose from and between 1 and 5 levels depending on the sector. Within reason, there is no maximum time limit to complete an NVQ; they are designed to be taken at a pace that suits the participant's needs.

Given the current state of unemployment across the world, gaining work experience while doing a degree, HN or NVQ has got to be a good thing!

Open University

A great resource for students in the UK is the Open University (OU) **www.open.ac.uk**. Its website offers a wide variety of options to students and tries to accommodate just about any kind of learning situation. It also has a wonderful study skills page that offers much helpful information, and it accommodates dyslexic students with its 'Services for Disabled Students'. The OU claims to support 9,000 students with learning difficulties (such as dyslexia).

The OU philosophy is to support and enable learning from anywhere, so you can study at home, while travelling, from abroad, or however you choose. This is a great way to catch up on education while working or raising children. Or you can pursue your credentials in a dedicated fashion until you are qualified. You build credits through a series of courses that are allocated different levels and points: you start with level 1 courses and work your way up, first to a foundation degree, and then to a full BA or BSc degree. You can even build your own curriculum up to a point with what is called the 'Open Degree'.

United States further education options

If you live in the United States, you have an unprecedented number of options for continuing education, higher education and career-specific training. The Division of Adult Education and Literacy (DAEL) promotes programmes to support basic education, secondary education and higher education for adults, as well as English language skills for immigrants and English language competency for those whose native language is English.

Learning is a lifelong pursuit and we are never finished

Most school districts in the US offer some kind of catch-up programme for adult learners to obtain the High School Diploma, or High School Diploma Equivalency, and colleges and schools routinely offer support for dyslexic learners. There is a wealth of online and onsite options for you to choose from. Start by looking on your local school district's website for adult and family education, Adult Basic Education (ABE) and Adult Secondary Education (ASE) programmes.

Some schools offer programmes that support parent and child learning together. This is a good environment for a parent to help a dyslexic learner, and often the reverse, for a child to help a parent who has dyslexia or a parent whose primary language is not English.

Vocational schools

There are a huge number of vocational schools in the United States and these can be a good way to get training fast for a wide variety of careers. Many offer career counselling and job placement assistance after a one-year (sometimes shorter) practical training. This approach can get young people into the workplace, making decent money and doing a job they enjoy, either for the rest of their lives, or as a stepping stone to a continuing education or degree programme.

In most areas of the country, there are options in almost any career field. If your child can dream of becoming it, he can most likely find a course that teaches it in one of numerous vocational institutions.

If you have the choice, look for one that has a recognised presence, such as Phoenix University or DeVry University, but do not rule out smaller schools if the vocational training offered is what you are looking for.

Online degrees

Most of the large, well-known institutions now offer some kind of continuing education online or online degree programme. It is almost impossible not to find a course that suits you. In fact, choices are so overwhelming that I recommend you take your time in researching the possibilities. If you find a programme that you might be interested in, I recommend using the 'contact us' link and try to establish a relationship with the admissions department in order to get more information before you sign up. Classes are not cheap and you want to make sure you sign up for something you really want to do.

One word of caution: look for a school that is accredited by the US Department of Education. You will also want to research what kinds of resources are offered to support dyslexic learners. Most offer some support, but some are better than others. As a rule of thumb, if you can't find information on the website, that college is probably not a good choice. A good example is the

University of Phoenix which advertises student disability services: **www.phoenix.edu/students/disability-services**.

Canadian further education options

Like the United States, Canada offers many options for finishing high school as an adult. The Mature High School Diploma[111] is a government-sponsored programme available to students over the age of 19 who have been out of school for at least six months.

Adult learning programmes in Canada make it easy to retake courses such as English and mathematics. You might just want to improve a grade for your college application, for example. Students are recommended to contact the college or university they are interested in attending to find out what their entrance requirements are.

Canada's different systems

The requirements for undertaking an Adult High School Diploma may vary from province to province, so it is best to check your local authority for options that may be available to you.

As an example, Alberta offers two types of diploma: the High School Equivalency Diploma and the Alberta High School Diploma[112]. The high school diploma is more academic than the equivalency diploma. Although both are accepted at most higher institutions, the high school diploma might be better accepted, because the equivalency diploma gives credit for maturity and life experiences over academic learning. So it is best to check with higher institutions that they will accept the Equivalency Diploma before you enrol.

Even though the high school diploma is considered better than an equivalency diploma, depending on the severity of dyslexia, an equivalency diploma is an attractive option due to the alternative routes available of accumulating credits and taking the General Education Development (GED) exam.

Most public school districts in Canada offer basic and supplemental academic classes to children and adults alike. For example, the Edmonton Public Schools Metro Continuing

Education office offers classes for children, youth and parents in basic English, academic subjects, technical subjects, business and home economics. It also offers English as a second language. You can choose a self-directed learning programme, where you work at your own pace, or an eight-week fast-track programme where you crunch through a lot of material in a short time.

You can expect major cities in Canada to have similar offerings to Edmonton's, including computer training, computer camps, youth programmes and continuing adult education programmes. Most also offer remote classes via the Internet.

For Canadians from other provinces, I recommend that you search on the Internet for education opportunities in your area. You also have access to a multitude of Canadian, US and international sites for online education through universities, colleges, and accredited institutions offering one-, two- and three-year certificates and diplomas. A good resource is the Community and Technical Colleges in Canada website,[113] which lists colleges and vocational schools throughout the country and in all the provinces.

Australian further education options

Whilst dyslexia is recognised in Australia under the Disability Discrimination Act 1992 (DDA) and under the Human Rights Commission, some schools still need to recognise dyslexia under the special needs section in the Education Act for additional funding as is the case in New South Wales.

In 2010, the Australian government published a report entitled *Helping People with Dyslexia: A National Action Agenda, from the Dyslexia Working Party*.[114] The report cites the work of Sir James Rose and the Rose Report in the UK, but its 19 recommendations to improve awareness of dyslexia and address educational support for dyslexic learners have yet to be implemented.

Until now, some schools and colleges have not been able to provide sufficient or any learning support. Knowing this can arm you to deal with the situation. The Australian people are passionate about supporting their learners and many organisations have their own resources for coping with dyslexia. You may wish to register your support for the national dyslexia campaign organisation (formed by Bris-bane Dys-lex-ics): **www.defydyslexia.com.au**.

The Central Institute of Technology offers nationally recognised courses for dyslexic students at its Perth campus.[115] The *Certificate I in Foundation Skills for Adults with Dyslexia* provides strategies for people with dyslexia to learn new coping skills and gain confidence in their English and maths skills. It also introduces technology aids to students. You can be evaluated for dyslexia at the campus if you are interested in enrolling.

There are many dyslexia associations in Australia: The SPEcific Learning Difficulties (SPELD) organisation is dedicated to helping children and adults with learning difficulties, especially dyslexia. Its centre in Victoria[116] offers support in literacy and maths, with specially trained teachers who understand how to address the challenges of dyslexic learners. They can also perform assessments. The Australian Dyslexia Association[117] is concerned with the well-being, identification and educational treatment of people with dyslexia. There are more associations in the **Appendix**.

The University of Adelaide offers Professional and Continuing Education (PCE) courses,[118] workshops and seminars to adults for a variety of educational purposes. Use this special programme to expand your vocational skills, retrain in new skills or improve your professional status in business or industry. For most courses there are no prerequisite qualifications.

Continuing education in Australia

Australia in general has many establishments for continuing education and serves adult educational needs very well. Centres for continuing secondary education offer adult education classes in both vocational and academic subjects for students aged 18 and older.

There are also supplemental education options for children between the ages of 9 and 12 and for children aged 15 and older who have left school. I would enquire with your local school to see what is available in your area.

EDucatioN Australia (EDNA)[119] is a nationwide network for education and training that includes government and non-government schools, vocational and technical training, and adult and community education. Through this network, you can find out about apprenticeships and specialised skills training and about skills that are in high demand (shortage skills) that you might be interested in training for.

Conclusion
Message to parents and children

I fell in love with the very thing I hated.

Vince Flynn, author[120]

Dear parents

If your child has difficulty learning, your encouragement and support will make all the difference. Your positive parenting skills can help your child emerge with a strong sense of self-worth and the determination to succeed. While learning difficulties do take their toll on family life, as so much more energy needs to be devoted to supporting our children, our attitude and approach can directly affect their outcome, as can the attitude and commitment of the school you choose.

Even though there will be times when you feel at your wits' end with worry, frustration or exhaustion, remember that you are not alone. With the right help, you can turn your situation around.

Dyslexia is just one of many challenges our children will face on their journey of life, so it is important to try to remain positive and encouraging and be realistic in our expectations and demands.

In the 21st century, we are better informed about dyslexia, and many of us adults have either been diagnosed with dyslexia or can at least relate to having learning challenges when we were at school. With this in mind, taking into consideration the inherited factors of dyslexia, if health specialists and nursery schools were to ask parents questions about inherited factors of dyslexia, or problems they had learning at school, then parents and teachers would know to look out for any of the signs of learning difficulties much earlier on. I believe that all nursery school and reception year teachers should be trained to recognise the early signs of dyslexia and any other learning difficulty.

Identifying children at risk of not acquiring literacy skills *before they start school* is easy. Between the ages of 0 and 3, our children have all the usual developmental milestone check-ups at the doctor's surgery. These check-ups are to ensure that the rate at which our child grows and changes physically, mentally, emotionally and socially is normal for his age. So why are we not looking for areas that hinder learning such as vision tracking, auditory processing, retained primitive reflexes, motor control and learning difficulties when children are at nursery school or when they first enter school?

Parents and educators have a role in ensuring that literacy failure is prevented, and we can make fostering high self-esteem in our children a top priority. I believe it is often possible to predict in Reception year whether a child will have future reading and writing problems. In my case, I instinctively felt that something was amiss when my children were about four/five years of age – even though I had never even heard of dyslexia, and I most certainly knew nothing about reading and writing difficulties.

Another area where nursery or primary schools can make a massive difference is in improving children's handwriting much earlier on. If nursery schools' and primary schools' handwriting policy included how children should hold their crayon, pencil and paintbrush correctly from the outset, it would reduce the number of children having handwriting difficulties and consequently underachieving academically in later years.

If you are not getting the support that your child needs from school, seek advice. Most schools and colleges around the world are finally acknowledging dyslexia and other learning difficulties and are trying hard to improve things. In some areas, improvement may still take some time, so you need to be proactive in advocating for your child, and getting what you want and rightly desire for him.

The sooner your child is put on a reading, writing, spelling, maths or self-esteem programme, the less likely it is that he will be playing catch-up at school and suffer the debilitating consequences of losing his self-esteem.

As we all know, our job as parents does not stop at being a nurse, taxi driver, chef, cleaner, counsellor and teacher. In many respects, we are destined to be our children's motivational coach too. We all need motivating and guidance. For example, an apprentice learns a new trade with a mentor, and actors or musicians generally need an agent. If you feel you do not have the skills necessary to coach a particular talent, perhaps you could ask a family member or friend to help.

We need to create opportunities for our children to be creative and discover and develop their talent

I believe that we are all born with creativity and the opportunity for talent. Both need to be nurtured to develop into skills.

If you have not yet discovered that your child has a learning difficulty, but you suspect that something is not right, listen to your gut feeling and ask for help as soon as possible. The earlier strategies and support are in place, the less likely it is that your child will fall behind at school or get demoralised, and the sooner he will begin to understand his strengths, develop coping strategies and use these to his advantage.

Early diagnosis and quick intervention are vital in improving the long-term outcomes for our children

I cannot emphasise enough the importance of having your child assessed, so that his learning can be appropriately managed. Children with undiagnosed and unmanaged dyslexia are more likely than their non-dyslexic peers to drop out of school, not go to college or university, become unemployed, be underemployed, or be imprisoned. Early diagnosis and quick intervention are vital in improving the long-term outcomes for our children. Making time for our talented children will ensure their success.

Remember there is help out there; you do not need to face it alone. There are many parents in similar situations, support groups and excellent professionals who understand and can help you and your child. Most important, *you need to nurture yourself*, so that you are mentally and emotionally strong enough to cope with supporting and motivating your child and are able to provide the unconditional love, sympathy and understanding he needs.

Dear children and teenagers

You know in your heart that you are amazing. You just know it! We were all born to make our mark in the world.

If you sense that something is not quite right, and it is bothering or upsetting you, share this with your parents, guardians, doctor or teachers. If you feel that you are capable of more or you cannot understand why things seem so tough at times, we can find ways to help you. If you can see a way of learning something in your way that would help you understand better, share it with your teacher. Your teacher is keen to find ways that will help you learn better.

When you are feeling down or not good enough, I urge you to write down or draw all the things you are good at. Try it! Sometimes it is easier to 'see' it written down. Draw or write down **everything**. Even list things you think are not that important (it's called brainstorming and every idea is valid). And just watch what begins to happen. You will begin to see **all the many, many things you are good at**. Some examples:

- I am good at caring for my dog and taking it for a walk every day
- I am good at being interested in wildlife and animals
- I am good at watching documentaries about our planet
- I am good at growing plants in the garden
- I am good at maths
- I am good at baking delicious chocolate cakes
- I am good at science and thinking up experiments

- I am good at constructing model aeroplanes
- I am good at improving the design of games I play with
- I am good at being a whiz with my skateboard
- I am good at riding my bike
- I am good at speaking foreign languages
- I am good at having a wild imagination for stories
- I am good at making up songs
- I am good at sculpting with clay
- I am good at thinking up amazing ideas
- I am good at taking great photos
- I am good at playing table tennis
- I am good at remembering historical events
- I am good at being kind and caring to others
- I am good at being a good friend
- I am good at geography
- I am good at saving money
- I am good at earning money at my local shop
- I am good at being stylish with my clothes
- I am good at being organised

Hang this list where you will see it every day so you can remind yourself of all the many things you are good at.

Also, draw pictures or write down a list of things you feel you are not good at, but remember to put: I am good at before everything you write or draw:

- **I am good at** having a messy room
- **I am good at** forgetting things sometimes
- **I am good at** being overwhelmed by too much information.

Sometimes, by turning our negatives into positives and developing coping strategies, we may even end up achieving in things that we think we are not so good at or that are in fact obstacles for us.

Having dyslexia, and finding reading, writing, spelling, speaking or remembering information hard, does not mean you cannot achieve your goals or become an author, motivational speaker or have a career that requires you to retain large amounts of information. For example, I was good at maths at school and not good at English; but I am a better teacher of English than I am of maths, as I can relate to the difficulties children have with English because I found it so hard.

With the help of a family member or friend, use your list to think about and write down all the opportunities you could pursue. There is a sample list below.

Turning Interests into Opportunities	
I am good at...	**Opportunities**
I am good at earning money	I can set up a club and teach other children how to turn their ideas into making money.
I am good at science	I can focus on an area of science that really interests me and become an expert in that field.
I am an expert biker and good at fixing bikes	I can set up a business selling and repairing bikes, or start a bikers' association or adventure travel company and organise events and tours.
I am good at being organised	I can think of innovative ways to help others who find organising themselves difficult and turn it into a great business idea.
I am good with people	I can set up a support group or a social group for anything I am interested in and get people to share their knowledge and stories to help one another

**By focusing on our talents and strengths,
our weaknesses seem to fade away**

You will see that you are good at many things. You may also begin to see a pattern of areas that interest you, and you could begin to focus your energy into developing that interest or talent. Then, show your list to someone who can help you investigate these ideas further and help you make these things happen. Perhaps one of these interests is your pathway in life?

If you feel that you are really good at something, however unusual it may be, tell your family. They want you to have a happy life, and they want you to try new things, so that you find what excites you and what makes you feel 'yippee'! But do not be disheartened if you try things and they do not work out. Do not give up – be determined! Sometimes, it takes lots and lots of attempts before we score that goal or win that certificate or finally don't burn our chocolate cake.

Do not give up, be determined! Remember, we are all talented at something. Maybe some people are born talented, but most of us develop interests into talents through **sheer hard work** and **perseverance**. By focusing on our talents and strengths, our weaknesses seem to fade away.

You only have to find **one** thing that really lights you up and makes you feel alive. It will take your mind off things that frustrate you, turn negative energy into positive energy and could even help you find your direction in life.

Discover your talent and follow your heart. Having dyslexia may even help you achieve your goal!

Carolina Fröhlich

Glossary

Access arrangements: Allow learners with special educational needs, disabilities or temporary injuries to access an assessment or examination. Access arrangements depend upon a learner's needs and are agreed before the assessment takes place and allow learners to show what they know and can do without changing the demands of the assessment; for example, 25% extra time; a reader, a scribe or use of technology.

Anomia: Part of the broader category of non-fluent aphasias, in which a person speaks hesitantly because of difficulty naming words and/or producing correct syntax.

Aphasia: Where the ability to understand language and to translate thoughts into words has been impaired by injury to the brain. Speaking, listening, reading or writing capabilities may be affected depending on the type of aphasia involved.

Apraxia: A neurologically-based motor speech disorder. A child with apraxia of speech has difficulty making the muscular movements necessary for making speech. Sometimes called verbal apraxia, developmental apraxia of speech or verbal dyspraxia.

Aptitude test: A test designed to measure general abilities and to predict future performance.

Attention: The process of focusing on certain stimuli while screening others out – how we actively process specific information.

Attention deficit disorder (ADD): Difficulty concentrating for long periods, planning ahead, following instructions and remembering things. Inattentive, but not hyperactive or impulsive. (Now comes under the umbrella of ADHD)

Attention-deficit/hyperactivity disorder (ADHD): May have difficulty maintaining attention because of a limited ability to concentrate; and/or with impulsive and hyperactive behaviour.

Attention span: The length of time a person can concentrate on a subject.

Auditory Processing Disorder (APD): APD interferes with the ability to interpret, process, analyse or make sense of information taken in through the ears. This is different from a hearing problem such as deafness, or being hard of hearing.

Autistic Spectrum Disorders (ASD): Subgroups within the spectrum of autism, a category of disability that significantly affects social interaction, verbal and non-verbal communication and educational performance.

Chronological age: The age of an individual in years. For example 7.7 represents an age of 7 years and 7 months.

Code of Practice: Guidelines that reflect the Education Act 2002 in the UK and inform both teachers and parents about good practice with regard to the special educational needs of children of school age.

Coping strategies: Methods or behavioural strategies that help an individual succeed in spite of learning or other difficulties.

Developmental Coordination Disorder (DCD): A broad term used to describe fine and gross motor skills or coordination difficulties.

Diagnostic tests: Tests of specific skills used to identify children's needs and to guide instruction.

Dysgraphia: Difficulty with handwriting caused by poor muscle sequencing or muscle memory in the fine motor skills required for efficient handwriting.

Dyslexia: 'A difficulty with words' that is primarily a difficulty learning and acquiring literacy skills (see full and official definition in chapter 'What is Dyslexia?').

Dysnomia: A noticeable difficulty in remembering names or recalling a word needed for oral or written language. Recall problems become dysnomia, which is a medical condition, when severe enough to interfere with daily life. Dysnomia is a lesser level of dysfunction than anomia.

Dyspraxia: This comes under the umbrella term 'Developmental Coordination Disorder' (DCD). A severely dyspraxic person may have trouble with gross and fine motor skills, perception, speech and language, and have poor organisational skills.

Early intervention: The process of intervening when a child or young person first shows signs of having difficulties.

Early intervention programmes: Compensatory programmes that target very young children at the greatest risk of school failure.

Educational psychological assessment: A clinical assessment using a selection of tests to establish academic potential.

Educational psychology: A scientific discipline that addresses the questions: 'Why do some students learn more than others?' and 'What can be done to improve their learning?'

Emotional and behavioural disorders: These are characterised by problems with learning, interpersonal relationships and control of feelings and behaviour.

Emotional intelligence (EI): An individual's ability to identify, assess, manage, understand and control the emotions of him/herself, of others and of groups.

Equality Act (2010): Anti-discrimination law in Great Britain that protects the rights of individuals and equal opportunity for all. Refer to p.8 Section 6 for learning difficulties.[121]

Expressive aphasia: Also known as motor aphasia, this condition hinders the ability to speak or express oneself and to say remembered words.

Expressive language: The production, spoken output and coding of language. A process of formulating ideas into words and sentences (speaking).

Fine motor skills: The smaller muscle groups of the body that enable functions such as writing, grasping small objects, typing, tying shoelaces and fastening clothing.

Full Scale IQ: An intelligence quotient made up of the average of four scores: Verbal Comprehension Index, Perceptual Reasoning Index, Working Memory Index and Processing Speed Index.

General Ability Index: An intelligence quotient made up of the average of two scores: Verbal Comprehension Index and Perceptual Reasoning Index.

Gifted: Gifted children have exceptional abilities in one or more subjects in the statutory school academic curriculum (except art and design, music and sports).

Gross motor skills: The larger muscle groups of the body that involve larger movements such as the arm, leg or foot or the entire body.

Individual Education Plan or Programme (IEP): A plan tailored to the needs of a specific child in order to address his/her particular difficulties. Sometimes known as a Learning Passport. Normally lasting for a term or six months, the IEP is then reviewed (subject to variation across schools). In the UK, it is not statutory. In the USA, it is a legal document.

Individuals with Disabilities Education Act (IDEA): A United States federal law that governs how public agencies and states provide early intervention, special education and related services to children with disabilities.

Intelligence: General aptitude for learning, often measured by ability to deal with abstractions and to solve problems.

Intelligence Quotient (IQ): An intelligence test score that should be near 100 for people of average intelligence.

Irlen Syndrome: See Scotopic sensitivity.

Kinaesthetic (tactile) learning: Learning by doing or physical activity (touch).

Learning Disability (LD): A lifelong condition, usually present from birth, that impedes the academic progress of people who are not mentally retarded or emotionally disturbed. It may not become apparent until a child fails to reach particular developmental milestones.

Learning styles/preferences: Orientation for approaching learning tasks and processing information in certain ways.

Loci method: Strategy for remembering lists by picturing items in familiar locations.

Long-term memory: Component of memory where large amounts of information can be stored for long periods.

Metacognition: Knowing about one's own learning and how one learns best ('thinking about thinking').

Metacognitive skills: The skills used by self-regulated learners who are able to reflect, understand and control their learning. Important for school and life.

Mind Mapping®: A diagram used to visually outline main ideas and connections between them.

Mnemonic: A method used to prompt the memory (memory link).

Motor aphasia: See Expressive aphasia.

Multiple Intelligences: Howard Gardner's theory of nine intelligences – a person's areas of ability.

Onset and Rime: Terms to describe phonological units of a spoken sylable. A syllable can normally be divided into two parts: the Onset is the initial consonant or consonant blend, and the Rime consists of the vowel and any final consonants. (e.g. 'swim' = 'sw-im')

Over-learning: Method of improving retention by practising new knowledge or skills until mastery/automaticity is achieved.

Perception: A person's interpretation of stimuli.

Perceptual Reasoning Index (PRI): This tests performance on tasks that require practical thinking and reasoning to do with pictures, designs and puzzles that do not require the use of words to reach solutions. Some tasks are against the clock and require accuracy and fluency.

Processing speed: The speed at which we process information. It generally refers to the varying speeds at which individuals are able to perform cognitive activities such as the recognition of simple stimuli.

Processing Speed Index (PSI): The ability to make judgements at speed by matching symbols, making decisions and transferring information.

Profound and Multiple Learning Difficulties (PMD): Describes children who have very complex needs that are normally met by special schools. Many have exceptionally poor communication skills.

Reading age: A reading test provides the reading age, and also enables the tester to discover the standard score and percentile point at which the child is reading, e.g. a reading age of 8.4 (expressed in years.months) would be the performance of an average child at 8 years and 4 months.

Receptive language: Comprehension of language. Receiving, understanding and 'decoding' language (listening and reading).

Remediation: Instruction given to students who have difficulty learning.

Rote learning: Memorisation of facts or associations.

Scaffolding: Techniques used to teach a specific aspect of basic skills. Teachers observe a child, identify his stage of learning and then provide support to help him reach the next stage. Support for learning and problem solving could be in the form of clues, reminders, encouragement, breaking the problem down into steps, providing an example, or anything else that allows the student to grow in independence as a learner.

Scotopic Sensitivity (Irlen) Syndrome:[122] Irlen Syndrome prevents many people from reading effectively and efficiently. The problems are caused by the way the brain interprets the visual information sent through the eyes. Individuals with Irlen Syndrome perceive reading material and/or their environment differently. They constantly make adaptations or compensate for their eye problems. The eyes are not the main source of the problem. Irlen lenses (colour tinted) or filters have been found to reduce or eliminate glare.

Self-actualisation: A person's desire to develop to his or her full potential.

Self-esteem: The value we each place on our own characteristics, abilities and behaviours.

Semantic memory: Part of long-term memory that stores facts and general knowledge.

Sensorimotor stage: Stage during which infants learn about their surroundings by using their senses and motor skills.

Sensory Processing Disorder (SPD): Difficulty processing (receiving and perceiving) sensory information through sight, sound, taste, smell, touch and movement (previously known as Sensory Integration Dysfunction).

Sequencing: The ability to remember, order or reconstruct information such as days of the week, months of the year, directions, lists, events or sounds. Most sequencing tasks have a memory element involved.

Short-term memory: Component of memory where limited amounts of information can be stored for a few seconds.

Spatial awareness: Understanding the relationship between yourself and the objects or people around you.

Special Educational Needs and Disability (SEND): Umbrella term that includes specific and global difficulties, permanent and temporary problems that affect the learning of children with academic, mental, emotional or physical disabilities.

Specific Learning Difficulties (SpLD): Children who operate in one or two areas at a level below that of their general functioning are said to be experiencing specific learning difficulties. There are many types: the one most commonly associated with this term is dyslexia.

Spelling age: A spelling test not only provides a spelling age, but also enables the tester to discover the standard score and percentile point at which a child is spelling. For example, a spelling age of 7.2 (expressed in years.months) would be the performance of an average child at 7 years and 2 months.

Talented: Talented children have exceptional abilities in art and design, music, sports, leadership skills or performing arts such as dance and drama.

Verbal Comprehension Index (VCI): An overall measure of the ability to reason verbally and also influenced by knowledge learned from one's environment.

Visual perception: The process of recognising, understanding, interpreting and organising visual information.

Visual Processing Disorder: A reduced ability to interpret or process information taken in through the eyes. It is not the same as having poor eyesight.

Waves 1, 2 and 3: Systematic intervention of tailored teaching provision in UK schools.

Working memory: Another term for short-term memory.

Working Memory Index (WMI): Formerly known as 'Freedom from Distractibility'. It requires short-term memory, receptive attention and concentration in order to achieve success. It is calculated through subtests: *Digit Span* – children are given sequences of numbers orally and asked to repeat them forwards and/or in reverse order. It provides a guide to levels of auditory memory and attention. *Letter–Number Sequencing* – children are given a series of numbers and letters and asked to provide them back to the examiner in a predetermined order. *Arithmetic* is a supplemental test consisting of orally administered arithmetic questions, which are timed.

Appendix A
Indicators of dyslexia by age

Indications of Dyslexia by Age
from the British Dyslexia Association[123]

Persisting factors

There are many persisting factors in dyslexia, which can appear from an early age and will still be noticeable when the child with dyslexia leaves school, including:

- Obvious 'good' and 'bad' days, for no apparent reason
- Confusion between directional words, e.g. up/down, in/out
- Difficulty with sequences, e.g. coloured bead sequence, later with days of the week or numbers
- A family history of dyslexia/reading difficulties

1. Pre-school

- Has persistent jumbled phrases, e.g. 'cobblers' club' for 'toddlers' club'
- Uses substitute words e.g. 'lampshade' for 'lamppost'
- Is unable to remember the label for known objects, e.g. 'table', 'chair'
- Has difficulty learning nursery rhymes and rhyming words, e.g. 'cat, mat, sat'
- Has later than expected speech development

Pre-school non-language indicators

- May have walked early but did not crawl – was a 'bottom shuffler' or 'tummy wriggler'
- Has persistent difficulties in getting dressed efficiently and putting shoes on the correct feet
- Enjoys being read to but shows no interest in letters or words

- Is often accused of not listening or paying attention
- Demonstrates excessive tripping, bumping into things and falling over
- Has difficulty with catching, kicking or throwing a ball, with hopping and/or skipping
- Has difficulty with clapping a simple rhythm

2. Primary school age

- Has particular difficulty with reading and spelling
- Puts letters and figures the wrong way round
- Has difficulty remembering tables, alphabet, formulae, etc.
- Leaves letters out of words or puts them in the wrong order
- Still occasionally confuses 'b' and 'd' and words such as 'no/on'
- Still needs to use fingers or marks on paper to make simple calculations
- Has poor concentration
- Has problems understanding what he has read
- Takes longer than average to do written work
- Has problems processing language at speed

Primary school age non-language indicators

- Has difficulty with tying shoelaces or tie, or with dressing
- Has difficulty telling left from right, order of days of the week, months of the year, etc.
- Surprises you because in other ways he is bright and alert
- Has a poor sense of direction and still confuses left and right
- Lacks confidence and has a poor self-image

3. *Aged 12 or over*

As for primary schools, plus:

- Still reads inaccurately
- Still has difficulties in spelling
- Needs to have instructions and telephone numbers repeated
- Gets 'tied up' using long words, e.g. 'preliminary', 'philosophical'
- Confuses places, times, dates
- Has difficulty with planning and writing essays
- Has difficulty processing complex language or long series of instructions at speed

Aged 12 or over non-language indicators:

- Has poor confidence and self-esteem
- Has areas of strength as well as weakness

Appendix B
Dyslexia and learning disabilities associations

UK and IRELAND

www.bdadyslexia.org.uk – Information for parents, adults WITH DYSLEXIA, and teachers. Worldwide and regional support groups

www.arkellcentre.org.uk – Helen Arkell Dyslexia Centre: courses for individuals with dyslexia, and teacher training. Provides assessments from educational psychologists, speech and language therapists and Helen Arkell trained assessors

www.dyslexiascotland.org.uk – Information for parents, educators and regional support groups

www.dyslexia.ie – Information for specific learning disabilities and dyslexia and regional support groups

www.dyslexiaaction.org.uk – Support for people with dyslexia and literacy difficulties

www.patoss-dyslexia.org – Professional association for teachers of students with specific learning difficulties

www.dyspraxiafoundation.org.uk – Supports children, families and adults with dyspraxia

www.addiss.co.uk – The National Attention Deficit Disorder Information and Support Service

www.hacsg.org.uk – Helps ADHD/hyperactive children and their families

www.autism.org.uk – Information and support for autism and Asperger syndrome

www.aspergerfoundation.org.uk – The Asperger Syndrome Foundation promotes awareness and understanding of Asperger Syndrome

www.nasen.org.uk – Promotes the education, training, advancement and development of special and additional support needs

www.ipsea.org.uk – IPSEA is a national charity providing free legally-based advice to families who have children with special educational needs

www.equalityhumanrights.com – A statutory body to protect, enforce and promote equality across the seven 'protected' grounds: age, disability, gender, race, religion and belief, sexual orientation and gender reassignment

EUROPE

www.eda-info.eu – European Dyslexia Association

USA

www.american-dyslexia-association.com – Information and teaching aids for people with dyslexia and dyscalculia
www.interdys.org – Information about current dyslexia research, publications, instructional technology, conferences and training programmes
www.ldonline.org – Information on learning disabilities, reading research, teacher tips, legal information and associated links
www.dyslexiafoundation.org – The Dyslexia Foundation Dyslexia Centers of America. Search under / Affiliates / Select State
www.smartkidswithld.org – Information for parents of children with learning disabilities (LD)
www.greatschools.org – Information to help parents and teachers understand learning difficulties

CANADA

www.ldac-acta.ca – Learning Disabilities Association of Canada: support groups across Canada
www.ldao.ca – Learning Disabilities Association Ontario
www.ldav.ca – Learning Disabilities Association Vancouver
idaontario.com – The International Dyslexia Association Ontario Branch
www.vidyslexiaassociation.com – Vancouver Island Dyslexia Association
www.ogtutors.com – Canadian Academy of Therapeutic Tutors
www.canlearn.ca – Government of Canada: grants, bursaries and scholarships
www.dyslexiaassociation.ca – Dyslexia Association Canada - Quebec

AUSTRALIA

www.dyslexiaassociation.org.au – Australia Dyslexia Assocation (ADA) based in Queensland, also in every state
www.dyslexiccentreaustralia.org.au – Dyslexia Centre in Western Australia
www.dyslexia-speld.com – DSF Literacy and Clinical Services
www.ldc.org.au – Learning Difficulties Coalition: individuals and parent support groups in NSW
www.dyslexia-testing.com.au – Information, support and assessments
www.everydaywithadhd.com.au – Links to ADHD groups in Australia and New Zealand
www.learningdifficulties.org.au – SSLDSG: Sutherland Shire Learning Disabilities Support Group – NSW
www.autismspectrum.org.au – Autism Spectrum Disorders (ASPECT), NSW
www.speldnsw.org.au – Specific learning difficulties NSW
www.ladswa.com.au – Learning and Attention Disorders in Western Australia (LADS) is a support agency for people with ADHD and associated conditions

NEW ZEALAND

www.dyslexiafoundation.org.nz – National organisation focused specifically on dyslexia
www.lbctnz.co.nz – Information on learning or behaviour difficulties
www.4d.org.nz – Dyslexia support for parents

SOUTH AFRICA

www.saaled.org.za – Southern African Association for Learning and Educational Difficulties

WORLDWIDE

dyslexia-international.org – Contacts for Ministries of Education worldwide and support groups. Search by country
www.dyslexia-international.org – Team of online consultants in literacy and reading difficulties

www.teachervision.fen.com – Teaching resources including special educational needs information
www.dyslexia.com – Davis Dyslexia Association International
www.adhd-federation.org –World Federation of ADHD
www.wdnf.info – International contacts worldwide

Appendix C
High learning potential and gifted websites

www.mensa.org.uk – The High IQ Society (UK)
www.ukmt.org.uk – United Kingdom Mathematics Trust
www.nace.co.uk – National Association for Able Children in Education
www.potentialplus.org.uk – Potential Plus UK
www.youthsporttrust.org – Youth Sport Trust
www.worldclassarena.org – World Class Arena
www.adifferentplace.org – A Different Place
www.hoagiesgifted.org – Hoagies Gifted Education
www.cty.jhu.edu – Johns Hopkins Center for Talented Youth
www.sengifted.org – Supporting Emotional Needs of Gifted
www.austega.com – Austega Gifted Resource Centre

Appendix D
Speech and language therapists and educational psychologists

UK

www.psychtesting.org.uk – Psychological testing centre
www.bps.org.uk – British Psychological Society. Search under/The Public icon Find a Psychologist
www.rcslt.org – The Royal College of Speech and Language Therapists. Search by post code under/Speech and Language therapy/Independent SLTs

EUROPE

www.cplol.eu – EU Speech and Language Therapists and Logopedists. (Comité Permanent de Liaison des Orthophonistes/Logopèdes de l'Union Européenne). Search under / Member Associations

USA

www.apa.org – American Psychological Association. Search under/Psychology Help Center
www.asha.org – The American Speech-Language-Hearing Association (ASHA). Search under/Public/Find a Professional

CANADA

www.cpa.ca – Canadian Psychological Association. Search under/Public/Provincial and Territorial Associations of Psychology
www.caslpa.ca – Canadian Authority of Speech-Language Pathologists and Audiologists. Search under/Consumers/Find a Professional

AUSTRALIA

www.psychology.org.au – Professional Association for
Psychologists. Search under/Community Information/Find a
Psychologist under Educational
www.speechpathologyaustralia.org.au – Speech Pathology
Australia. Search under/Information for the Public

NEW ZEALAND

www.psychology.org.nz – Professional Association for
Psychologists. Search under/Find a Psychologist
www.speechtherapy.org.nz – New Zealand Speech Therapy
Association. (NZSTA). Search under/Information for Families

SOUTH AFRICA

www.psyssa.com – South African Psychological Society
(PsySSA). Search under/Search for a Psychologist
www.saslha.co.za – Speech-Language Therapists and
Audiologists in South Africa. Search under/For the Public/Find a
Professional (by location)

WORLDWIDE

www.nepes.eu – Network of Educational Psychologists in the
Education System. Search under/Across Europe/National
Associations worldwide

Appendix E
Schools, colleges and universities with SEN/D provision worldwide

UK and IRELAND

www.crested.org.uk – Register of schools that help children with specific learning difficulties (dyslexia)
www.gettherightschool.co.uk – Every aspect of education, including SEN and bullying
www.goodschoolsguide.co.uk – Details all schools in the UK: State and Independent schools with SEN provision, plus special schools
www.learndirect.co.uk – 16+ information about courses, business, non-traditional forms of learning
www.gov.uk – Government Disabled Students' Allowances (DSA) provide extra financial help for students in further or higher education with a disability or specific learning difficulty. Search under Education and Learning
www.gov.uk – Access to Work – practical help at work including technology and equipment. Under Disabled People/Employment support/Work schemes and programmes
www.prospects.ac.uk – University careers advice; courses; job markets
www.dyslexia.ie – Search under Schools and Support or www.dyslexia.ie/schoolsup.htm
www.education.ie – Government Department of Education. Listings of Primary and Special schools by county.

USA

www.iser.com – ISER (Internet Special Education Resources) lists schools by State
www.gow.org – The GOW School in New York. Search under LD-friendly Colleges (US and Canada)
www.clas.ufl.edu/au – Index of American Universities

www.college-scholarships.com – Colleges and universities that support students with learning disabilities. Under Colleges with programmes for learning disabled

www.fairtest.org – Schools that do not use SAT or ACT scores for admitting substantial numbers of students into bachelor degree programmes

CANADA

www.ourkids.net/school – Our Kids Go To School: private-school search by name or postal code

www.gov.bc.ca/bced/ – Each State has its own Ministry of Education website; the one listed is for British Columbia. Search under For Parents/Schooling Options for My Child

www.schoolfinder.com – By university, college or career

www.canadian-universities.net – A guide to Canadian universities, community colleges, career colleges and jobs in Canada

www.canlearn.ca – Government of Canada: grants, bursaries and scholarships

AUSTRALIA

www.schools.nsw.edu.au – Each state has its own Public Schools' website; the one listed is for NSW. Search under Supporting Students/Disability Programs/ (support classes in regular schools)

www.australian-universities.com – By city and state. Link to home page of university and search 'special needs' or 'dyslexia' for provision

NEW ZEALAND

www.minedu.govt.nz – Ministry of Education for New Zealand. Search under Parents

MALAYSIA

www.learn4good.com/great_schools/children_schools_malaysia.htm – Search by country

SOUTH AFRICA

www.schoolguide.co.za – Alphabetical list of special education schools 3–21 years. Excellent information and web links to the schools
www.isasa.org – Independent Schools Association of Southern Africa. Search under Schools
www.saschools.co.za – South African Web Enabled Schools (State and Private). Search under Schools Directory

WORLDWIDE

www.findaschool.org – Links to higher education facilities worldwide
www.learn4good.com – Search by any country around the world

Appendix F
Publishers and suppliers of special education resources

UK and IRELAND

www.crossboweducation.co.uk – Visual stress resources, multisensory teaching resources, behaviour management, handwriting aids
www.smartkids.co.uk – Large selection of multisensory resources
www.inclusive.co.uk – Hardware and software to help all learners
www.bdatech.org – British Dyslexia Association technology resources
www.learningspaceni.co.uk – Educational resources, games and software
www.r-e-m.co.uk – Educational software and teaching resources
www.risingstars-uk.com – Books, teaching resources and software
www.rm.com – Provider of ICT education software
www.ldalearning.com – Traditional resources
www.adapt-it.org.uk – Hardware and software
www.aidis.org – Resources to help disabled people communicate through technology
www.happypuzzle.co.uk – Resources for children with special educational needs such as dyslexia and dyspraxia, as well as gifted and talented children
www.cricksoft.com – Reading and writing software for home use

NORTH AMERICA and CANADA

www.target.com – Learning toys. Melissa and Doug Magnetic Responsibility Chart
www.turningpointtechnology.com – Equipment, software, hardware for children and adults with learning disabilities

www.bloomingkids.com – Software for teaching children with special needs
www.donjohnston.com – Special needs resources, intervention solutions and assistive technology programmes

Appendix G
Revision websites

www.bbc.co.uk/schools/bitesize – All subjects for all ages
www.cgpbooks.co.uk – CPG study guides for older learners
www.philipallan.co.uk – Philip Allan revision guides and ready-made flash cards for older learners
www.s-cool.co.uk – Free GCSE and A-level revision material by subject. Tips about passing exams, and careers advice
www.podcastrevision.co.uk – Free downloadable podcasts of all GCSE English language and literature. Excellent explanations of poems
www.universalteacher.org.uk – Free GCSE and A-Level English language and literature for revising poems, books, AQA anthology. It has in-depth commentaries on all poems in the current anthology
getrevising.co.uk/resources/level/a_ib – International Baccalaureate revision site
https://global.oup.com/education/?region=international – International revision books for IB PYP, IB MYP, iGCSE and IB

Appendix H
Motivation and revision charts

Personal Goal _____

Mini Targets to reach my goal	Mon	Tues	Wed	Thurs	Fri	Sat	Sun	Achieved
1.								
2.								
3.								
4.								
5.								

Do something fun every day!

Reading Reward Chart

Book Title _____

Week Commencing	Mon	Tue	Wed	Thurs	Fri	Sat	Sun	Reward

I will read 20 minutes every day. ☺ Signed _____

Getting Organised – Home

Things to remember at home	Mon	Tues	Wed	Thurs	Fri	Sat	Sun
Date							

Getting Organised – School

Things to remember for school	Mon	Tues	Wed	Thurs	Fri	Sat	Sun
Date							

Performance Chart

Excellent Performance ☺ ☹	Mon	Tues	Wed	Thurs	Fri	Sat	Sun
Date							

My reward							

Revision Timetable Chart

Revise mornings only Date	Mon	Tue	Wed	Thurs	Fri	Sat	Sun
Revision – 30 mins	Eng	History	French	Biology	Chemistry		F
			10 mins break				A
Revision – 30 mins	Eng	History	French	Biology	Chemistry		M
			10 mins break				I
Revision – 30 mins	Maths	Geog	RS	Physics	Latin		L
			20 mins snack break				Y
Revision – 30 mins	Maths	Geog	RS	Physics	Latin		
			10 mins break				T
Revision Recap – 30 mins	Eng	History	French	Biology	Chemistry		I
			10 mins break				M
Revision Recap – 30 mins	Maths	Geog	RS	Physics	Latin		E
Afternoons	FUN	FUN	FUN	FUN	FUN		

References

Baddeley AD and Hitch GJL (1974) Working Memory. In Bower GA (ed.) *The Psychology of Learning and Motivation: Advances in Research and Theory.* New York: Academic Press, pages 47–89.

Bolles EB (1988) Remembering and Forgetting: Inquiries into the Nature of Memory. New York: Walker.

Bond J, Coltheart M, Connell T, Firth N, Hardy M, Nayton M, Shaw J and Weeks A (2010) Helping People with Dyslexia: A National Action Agenda: Report to the Hon Bill Shorten, Parliamentary Secretary for Disabilities and Children's Services, from the Dyslexia Working Party. www.dysletffxiaaustralia .com.au/DYSWP.pdf (21 July 2010).

Bradford J (2008) Using Multisensory Teaching Methods, Dyslexia Online Magazine, 30. http://beckyhinze.pbworks.com /f/Using+multisensory.docx (accessed 15 October 2013).

British Medical Association (2005) Preventing childhood obesity. www.iaso.org/site_media/uploads/Preventing_childhood_obesi ty_2005.pdf (accessed 15 October 2013)

Buttriss J and Callander A (2008) *The A-Z of Special Needs: For Every Teacher.* London: Optimus Education.

Clark C (2007) Why Families Matter to Literacy: A Brief Research Review. London: National Literacy Trust.

Clark C (2009) *Why Fathers Matter to their Children's Literacy.* London: National Literacy Trust.

Cline S and Schwartz D (1999) *Diverse Populations of Gifted Children.* Upper Saddle River, NJ: Merrill.

Cope, Natalie, Harold, Denise, Hill, Gary, Moskvina, Valentina, Stevenson, Jim, Holmans, Peter, Owen, Michael J., O'Donovan, Michael C. and Julie, Williams (2005) Strong evidence KIAA0319 on chromosome 6p is a susceptibility gene for developmental dyslexia. *American Journal of Human Genetics,* 76, (4), 581–591.

Davis RD (1997) The Gift of Dyslexia: Why Some of the Brightest People Can't Read and How They Can Learn. London: Souvenir Press.

Dowell B (2003) Secret of the Super Successful... They're Dyslexic, Times Online, 5 October. www.thetimes.co.uk/tto/health/article1880462.ece (accessed 15 October 2013).

Faiers R (ed.) (1989) This England's Book of Parlour Poetry. Cheltenham: This England Books.

Flouri E and Buchanan A (2004) Early Father's and Mother's Involvement and Child's Later Educational Outcomes, British Journal of Educational Psychology, 74,141–153.

Gardner H (1983) Frames of Mind: The Theory of Multiple Intelligences. New York: Basic.

Garner R (2005) 'Humor, Analogy and Metaphor: H.A.M. It Up in Teaching', Radical Pedagogy, 6 (2): 1. www.radicalpeda gogy.org/radicalpedagogy94/Humor,_Analogy,_and_Metaph or__H.A.M._it_up_in_Teaching.html (21 July 2010).

Glenn R (2002) Brain Research: Practical Applications for the Classroom, Teaching for Excellence, 21 (6): 1–2.

Goleman D (1995) Emotional Intelligence: Why It Can Matter More Than IQ. London: Bloomsbury.

Gottman J (1998) Raising an Emotionally Intelligent Child: The Heart of Parenting. New York: Simon and Schuster.

Jordan-Black J (2005) The Effects of the Primary Movement Programme on the Academic Performance of Children Attending Ordinary Primary School, Journal of Research in Special Educational Needs 5(3): 101–111.

Krupska M and Klein C (1995) Demystifying Dyslexia. London: London Language and Literacy Unit, South Bank University.

Lyman D (1986) Making the Words Stand Still. Austin, TX: Houghton Mifflin.

Lyon GR (1996) State of Research. In Cramer S and Ellis W (eds) *Learning Disabilities: Lifelong Issues.* Baltimore, MD: Brooks Publishing, pages 3–61.

Maslow, AH (1943) 'Theory of Human Motivation', *Psychological Review* 50(4): 370–96.

Mastropieri MA and Scruggs TE (2000) *The Inclusive Classroom: Strategies for Effective Teaching.* Columbus, OH: Prentice Hall.

McPhillips M, Hepper PG, Mulhern G. (2000) Effects of replicating primary-reflex movements on specific reading difficulties in children: a randomised, double-blind, controlled trial. *The Lancet* 2000; 355:537.

McKown BA and Barnett CL (2007) *Improving Reading Comprehension through Higher-Order Thinking Skills*, MA thesis, Chicago, IL: Saint Xavier University. (ERIC Document Reproduction Service No. ED496222).

Morrison MK (2008) Using Humor to Maximize Learning: The Links between Positive Emotions and Education. Lanham, MD: Rowman and Littlefield Education.

Muccillo A (2008) Tapping for Kids: A Children's Guide to Emotional Freedom Technique. Eastbourne: Dragonrising.

Nicholson W (2000) *The Wind Singer.* London: Mammoth.

Ormrod JE (2007) *Educational Psychology: Developing Learners.* Upper Saddle River, NJ: Prentice Hall.

Puder C (2003) The Healthful Effects of Laughter, *The International Child and Youth Care Network*, 55 (August). www.cyc-net.org/cyc-online/cycol-0803-humour.html (21 July 2010).

Richardson AJ and Wilmer J (2001) Association between Fatty Acid Symptoms and Dyslexic and ADHD Characteristics in Normal College Students. Paper presented at *British Dyslexia Association International Conference*, University of York, April.

Robinson FP (ed.) (1970) *Effective Study.* New York: Harper & Row.

Rose J (2006) *Independent Review of the Teaching of Early Reading.* London: Department for Education and Skills. http://webarchive.nationalarchives.gov.uk/20100526143644/http:/standards.dcsf.gov.uk/phonics/report.pdf (accessed 15 October 2013).

Silverman L (2002) Poor Handwriting: A Major Cause of Underachievement. In Silverman L (ed.) *Upside-Down Brilliance: The Visual Spatial Learner.* Denver, CO: DeLeon.

Society for Neuroscience (2004) *Dyslexia: Making a Difference Today.* Washington, DC: Society for Neuroscience. www.techrepublic.com/resource-library/whitepapers/dyslexia-making-a-difference-today/ (15 October 2013).

Stein J (2006) *Dietary Supplements, Myth or Magic: The Neural Basis of Dyslexia.* Oxford: University of Oxford. http://visionhelp.files.wordpress.com/2010/12/john-stein-lecture-on-visual-basisi-of-reading-impairment.pdf (accessed 15 October 2013).

Thomson M (2007) *Dyslexia and Music.* Stirling: Dyslexia Scotland. http://dyslexicadvantage.wikispaces.com/file/view/DyslexiaandMusic.pdf (21 July 2010).

Tulip Financial Research Ltd ([n.d.]) *Britain's Millionaires: The Private Investment Powerhouse.* London: Tulip Financial Research Ltd. http://website.lineone.net/~john.clemens/reports.html (accessed 15 October 2013).

Unicef (2007) *Implementation Handbook for the Convention on the Rights of the Child: Article 31.* New York: Unicef. http://article31.ipaworld.org/wp-content/uploads/2009/10/Article31-2007edition.pdf (21 July 2010).

Walberg HJ and Tsai S-L (1983) Matthew Effects in Education, *American Educational Research Journal* 20 (3): 359–373.

Webb J and Latimer D (1993) ADHD and Children Who Are Gifted, *ERIC Digest,* 522.

Webb-Michael B (1995) The Importance of Stories in the Act of Caring, *Pastoral Psychology*, 43 (3): 215–225.

Wenner M (2009) The Serious Need for Play, *Scientific American*, February. www.scientificamerican.com/article.cfm?id=the-serious-need-for-play (21 July 2010).

Yeats WB (1935/1986) *The Autobiography of William Butler Yeats*. London: Macmillan.

Endnotes

1   Tulip Financial Research Ltd
    ([n.d.])
2   Dowell (2003)
3   www.virgin.com (MP3 file
    accessed 29 July 2013)
4   I use the UK system
    throughout the book.
    Reception is known in some
    countries as kindergarten.
    Confusingly, Year 1 (age 5–6)
    is also sometimes known as
    kindergarten
5   Grade 1 in the US
6   usatoday30.usatoday
    .com/news/health/spotlight/2
    001-05-22-brockovich-
    dyslexia.htm (accessed 2
    August 2013)
7   www.authorsden.com/
    visit/viewshortstory.asp?id=107
    67 (accessed 31 July 2013)
8   Society for Neuroscience
    (2004)
9   www.bdadyslexia.org.uk/
    about-dyslexia/faq.html
    (accessed 24 July 2013)
10 www.interdys.org/FAQ.htm
    (accessed 3 December 2012)
11 Davis (1997, pp 3–5)
12 www.bennettstrahan.
    com/article_apbenke.html
    (accessed 29 July 2013)
13 Genecards, Listing of Disease
    Genes www.genecards.org
    (accessed 14 October 2012)
14 www.ncbi.nlm.nih.gov/
    pmc/articles/PMC1199296/
    Cope, Natalie, Harold,
    Denise, Hill, Gary, Moskvina,
    Valentina, Stevenson, Jim,
    Holmans, Peter, Owen,
    Michael J., O'Donovan,
    Michael C. and Julie, Williams
    (2005, pp581-591) (accessed
    14 October 2012)
15 www.ncbi.nlm.nih.gov/
    pubmed/22750057Variants in
    the DYX2 locus are associated
    with altered brain activation
    in reading-related brain
    regions in subjects with
    reading disability. 2012 Oct
    15;63(1):148-56. (accessed 14
    October 2012)
16 Genetics of Dyslexia. Dyslexic
    Research Trust
    www.dyslexic.org.uk/research
    -genetics.html (accessed 14
    October 2012)
17 http://cordis.europa.eu/docu
    ments/documentlibrary/12248
    7781EN6.pdf (accessed 15
    October 2013) (accessed 9
    December 2012)
18 www.irlen.org.uk (accessed
    17 July 2013)
19 Stein (2006)
20 www.gosh.nhs.uk/medical-
    conditions/clinical-
    specialties/audiological-
    medicine-information-for-
    parents-and-visitors/
    (accessed 3 December 2012)
21 www.uhs.nhs.uk/Media/
    Controlleddocuments/Patient
    information/Earnoseandthroa
    t/Auditoryprocessing-
    patientinformation.pdf
    (accessed 3 December 2012)
22 www.rhythmicmovement
    training.com (accessed 14
    December 2012)

23 www.mydyslexiasolutions
    .com/FamousDyslexics.html
    (accessed 7 December 2012)
24 www.dyspraxiafoundation
    .org.uk/services/dys_glance.p
    hp (Permission granted.
    Accessed 16 August 2013)
25 Silverman (2002)
26 Silverman (2002)
27 apache2-cabo.guilder
    .dreamhost.com/PDF_files/Arti
    cles Archive/vsl/v37.pdf
    (accessed 3 August 2013)
28 www.aboutdyscalculia.org
    (Permission granted to
    reproduce characteristics.
    Accessed 16 August 2013)
29 www.speech-language-
    therapy.com/ (accessed 17
    July 2013)
30 www.quotes.net/ quote/6798
    (accessed 4 November 2012)
31 www.bucks.edu/~specpop/
    memory.htm (accessed 7
    December 2012)
32 Baddeley and Hitch (1974)
33 www.psychologistworld.com/
    memory/millermagicnumber
    .php (accessed 17 July 2013)
34 The brain from top to bottom;
    different types of long-term
    memory thebrain.mcgill
    .ca/flash/a/a_07/a_07_p/a_0
    7_p_tra/a_07_p_tra.html - 3
    (accessed 17 July 2013)
35 Children's under-
    achievement could be down
    to poor working memory, Feb
    2008,
    www.physorg.com/news1234
    04466.html (accessed 17 July
    2013)
36 Kendra Van Wagner,
    Forgetting: when memory fails
    psychology.about.com/od/
    cognitivepsychology/p/forgetti
    ng.htm (accessed 17 July 2013)
37 See Memory and its Role in
    Overcoming Dyslexia by Jan
    Strydom and Susan Du Plessis,
    www.audiblox2000.com/
    dyslexia_dyslexic/dyslexia009.
    htm (accessed 18 July 2013).
    They quote Donald Lyman's
    book Making the Words Stand
    Still (Lyman, 1986).
38 How To Remember Things.
    www.psychologytoday.
    com/blog/happiness-in-
    world/200911/how-remem ber-
    things www.scielo.br/
    pdf/bjmbr/v41n6/7019.pdf
    (accessed 18 July 2013)
39 http://thinkbuzan.com/
    (accessed 15 October 2013)
40 http://thinkbuzan.com/
    (accessed 15 October 2013)
41 www.brainyquote.com/
    quotes/authors/b/bruce_jenn
    er.html (accessed 15 October
    2013)
42 Goleman (1995)
43 Webb-Michael (1995)
44 Haugen, D ([2003]) Telling
    History: Scope and Purpose,
    www.wcdd.com/wc/
    proposals/thprop/thscope
    .html (accessed 23 June 2013)
45 www.bbc.co.uk/ouch/
    features/high_achieving_dysl
    exics.shtml (accessed 1
    August 2013)
46 Maslow (1943)
47 Richardson and Wilmer
    (2001), cited in
    www.foodforthe
    brain.org/content.asp?
    id_Content=1636 (accessed
    17 July 2013)
48 www.foodforthebrain.org
    (accessed 17 July 2013)
49 McGovern, M.K. (2005) The
    Effects of Exercise on the
    Brain, serendip.brynmawr

.edu/bb/neuro/neuro05/web
2/mmcgovern.html
(accessed 21 July 2013)
50 Unicef (2007)
51 Thomas: *Raising Smart and
Socially Well-Adjusted
Children*, www.open
education.net/2009/03/04/rai
sing-smart-and-socially-well-
adjusted-children (accessed
21 July 2010)
52 dyslexia.yale.edu/benacerraf
.html (accessed 31 July 2013)
53 Nicholson (2000)
54 www.potentialplusuk.org/
new_schools_main.php?cont
entid=441&webid=425#.ULiqC
awj7yA (Permission granted to
reproduce characteristics.
Accessed 31 July 2013)
55 Gardner (1983)
56 www.potentialplusuk.org/
new_schools_main.php?cont
entid=451&webid=426#.ULifN
Kwj7yA (accessed 7 February
2013)
57 www.vark-learn.com/english
/page.asp?p=biography
(accessed 8 December 2012)
58 Anonymous author. Quoted
from Faiers (1989)
59 www.visualspatial.org/
files/idvsls.pdf (accessed 9
December 2010)
60 sciencecareers.science
mag.org/career_magazine/pr
evious_issues/articles/2012_05
_11/caredit.a1200052
(accessed 31 July 2013)
61 Rose (2009)
62 www.al.com/specialreport/
huntsvilletimes/index.ssf?/hunt
svilletimes/dyslexia/content/d
ys3.html (accessed 27 July
2013)
63 Example screening tests:
available from Lucid

Research and Smart Cat
Learning (from +4 years old)
or AmIDyslexic (+16 years)
64 sdep.bps.org.uk/sdep/
publications/assessment.cfm
(Permission granted.
Accessed 21 January 2013)
65 Access Arrangements.
http://www.jcq.org.uk
(accessed 1 March 2012)
66 www.ldonline.org/article/High
_School_Graduation_Require
ments_and_Students_with_Dis
abilities (accessed 11 May
2012)
67 www.mensa.org.uk/iq-levels/
(accessed 29 November
2012)
68 www.dailymail.co.uk/health/
article-49795/Me-health-Steve-
Redgrave.html (accessed 1
Aug 2013)
69 www.examiner.com/article/
former-us-vice-president-
governor-of-ny-nelson-
rockefeller-had-adhd
(accessed 2 August 2013)
70 www.hwtears.com
71 www.kber.co.uk/hfw30.htm
72 www.franklin.com
73 www.gingersoftware.com
74 www.wordshark.co.uk
75 www.wordshark.co.uk
76 www.gailgodwin.com
(accessed 30 July 2013)
77 www.apnewsarchive.com/
1990/People-in-the-News/id-
e60aa5ac1dfba6ddd1a
63155d417af56 (accessed 30
July 2013)
78 McKown and Barnett (2007)
79 Bradford (2008)
80 thephotosociety.org/ blog/to-
light-a-fire/ (accessed 2
August 2013)
81 Clark (2009)

82 Flouri and Buchanan (2004), quoted in Clark (2009)

83 Clark (2007)

84 www.waterstones.com/wat/images/special/mag/waterstones_dyslexia_action_guide.pdf (accessed 21 July 2013)

85 www.oup.com/oxed/primary/oxfordreadingtree (accessed 9 November 2012)

86 http://thinkexist.com/quotation/do_not_worry_about_your_problems_with_mathematics/15457.html (accessed 15 October 2013)

87 www.goodreads.com/quotes/show/9680 (accessed 8 December 2012)

88 2005 CU Special Year in Art and Mathematics, http://plus.maths.org/content/artmathx (accessed 15 October 2013)

89 Thomson (2007)

90 Can Music Really Make You Smarter? www.musicaladvantage.com/ smarter.htm (accessed 21 July 2013)

91 http://gseis.ucla.edu/people/catterall(accessed 15 October 2013)

92 Choi, C.Q. (2007) *Playing Music Makes You Smart*, March 2007, www.livescience.com/health/070319_music_brainstem.html (accessed 24 July 2013)

93 Music Lessons Boost Brain Power, *Fox News*, November 2009 www.foxnews.com/scitech/2009/11/06/music-lessons-boost-brain-power (accessed 24 July 2013)

94 www.thrass.co.uk (accessed 21 July 2012)

95 Don Campbell, The Mozart Effect®, and the Mozart Effect for Children, www.mozarteffect.com (accessed 21 July 2012)

96 www.suzukiassociation.org (accessed 21 July 2012)

97 www.brainyquote.com/quotes/authors/b/bruce_jenner.html (accessed 15 October 2013)

98 www.xtraordinarypeople.com/celebrity/3/Tom-Cruise/ (accessed 2 August 2013)

99 Brain Gym was created by Paul Dennison PhD; see his website at: www.braingym.org or www.braingym.com and the UK Brain Gym site at www.braingym.org.uk (accessed 17 July 2012)

100 Jordan-Black (2005). See also www.primarymovement.org (accessed 2 August 2013)

101 www.primarymovement.org/research/extract2.html (accessed 31 July 2013)

102 Robinson (1970)

103 www.guardian.co.uk/world/2009/apr/18/whoopi-goldberg-saturday-interview (accessed 8 December 2012)

104 www.dys-add.com/symptoms.html (accessed 8 December 2012)

105 www.prospects.ac.uk (accessed 5 September 2013)

106 www.learndirect.co.uk (accessed 5 September 2013)

107 www.ucas.ac.uk (accessed 5 September 2013)

108 www.gov.uk/disabled-students-allowances-dsas/overview (accessed 25 August 2013)

109 www.edexcel.com/quals/highernationals10/Pages/default.aspx (accessed 5 September 2013)

[110] www.edexcel.com/
(accessed 15 October2013)

[111] www.edu.gov.mb.ca/k12/
policy/mat_student.html
(accessed 6 September 2013)

[112] www.adlc.ca/content/
view/35/36 (accessed 11
November 2012)

[113] www.cset.sp.utoledo.edu/
canctcol.html (accessed
11 November 2012)

[114] Bond *et al.* (2010)
(http://www.dyslexiaaustralia.
com.au/DYSWP.pdf)

[115] www.central.wa.edu.au
(accessed 5 September 2013)

[116] www.speldvic.org.au
(accessed 6 September 2013)

[117] dyslexiaassociation.org.au/
(accessed 6 September 2013)

[118] www.adelaide.edu.au/pce/
(accessed 11 November
2012)

[119] apps-new.edna.edu.au/
edna_retired/edna/go.html
(accessed 6 September 2013)

[120] www.examiner.com/
education-in-national/best-
selling-author-vince-flynn-
feels-his-dyslexia-is-a-gift
(accessed 8 December 2012)

[121] odi.dwp.gov.uk/docs/
wor/new/ea-guide.pdf
(accessed 24 July 2013)

[122] www.irlen.org.uk (accessed
21 July 2013)

[123] www.bdadyslexia.org.uk/
about-dyslexia/parents/
indications-of-dyslexia.html
(Permission granted.
Accessed 7 February 2013)

The publisher accepts no
responsibility for the persistence or
accuracy of URLs referred to in
this publication and does not
guarantee that any content on
such websites is or will remain
accurate or appropriate.

Index

Note: References in **bold** are to the Glossary.

You can contact Carolina via her website

www.carolinafrohlich.co.uk

*You can also find more information,
news of future appearances and books,
as well as links from the book to the
resources found here.*

33323930R00263

Made in the USA
Lexington, KY
21 June 2014